Thai Massage

MANUAL

Thai Massage
MANUAL

*Natural therapy for
flexibility, relaxation
and energy balance*

MARIA MERCATI

Photography by
Sue Atkinson

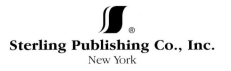

Sterling Publishing Co., Inc.
New York

To my loving family: Trevor, Gisela, Gina, Graham and Danella.

Library of Congress
Cataloging-in-Publication Data Available

10 9 8 7 6 5 4 3 2 1

Published in 1998 by Sterling Publishing Company, Inc.
387 Park Avenue South, New York, N.Y. 10016

Distributed in Canada by Sterling Publishing
c/o Canadian Manda Group, One Atlantic Avenue, Suite 105
Toronto, Ontario, Canada M6K 3E7

Sterling ISBN 0-8069-1755-5

AN EDDISON • SADD EDITION
Edited, designed and produced by
Eddison Sadd Editions Limited
St Chad's House
148 King's Cross Road
London WC1X 9DH

Phototypeset in Garamond ITC and Humanist 777 BT using QuarkXpress on Apple Macintosh
Origination by Bright Arts PTE, Singapore
Printed and bound by Shenzhen Donnelley Bright Sun, China

CONTENTS

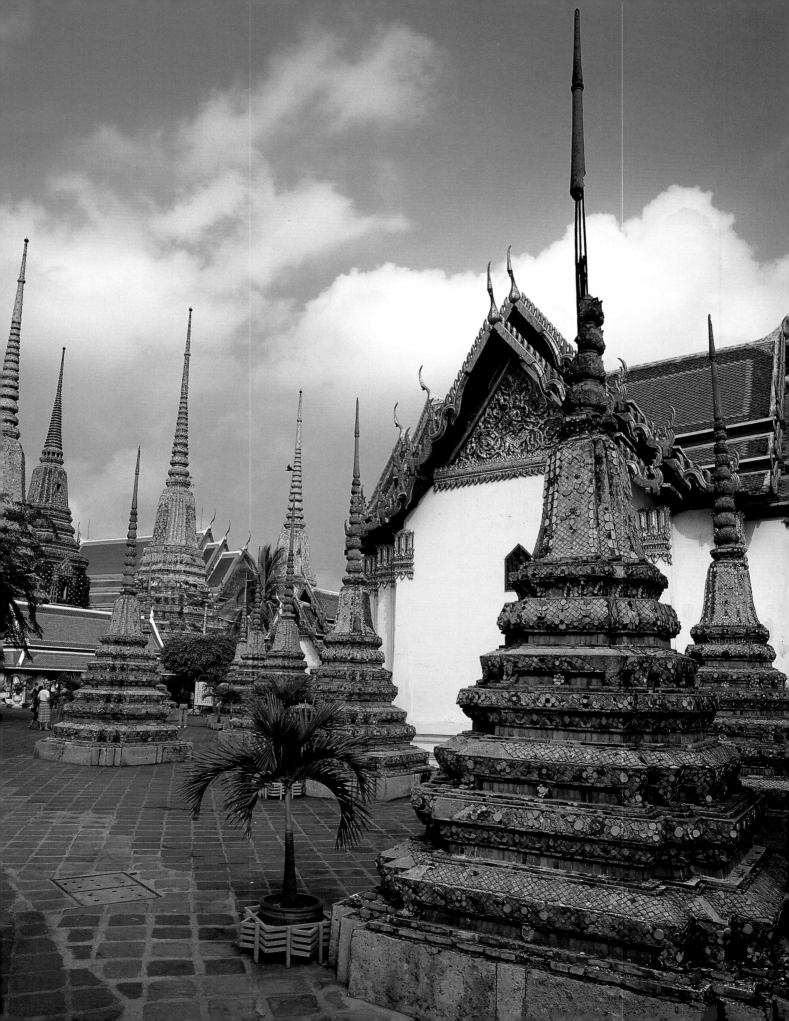

A NOTE FROM THE AUTHOR

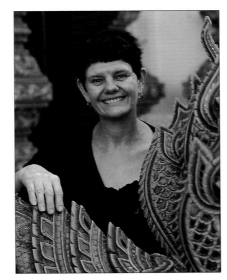

During the early 1980s I lived with my family in Indonesia for four years. It was here that I first discovered the healing massage. Extensive travels in south-east Asia eventually brought me to Thailand where I began treatment and training in traditional Thai massage. Since childhood I had suffered from Perthes disease – a chronic degenerative condition of the hip joint – and the wonderful stretching effects of Thai massage seemed like a miracle cure. Flexibility in my legs, including the affected joint, improved enormously and Thai massage has continued to enhance the flexibility and mobility of my body to the present day. However, Thai massage not only balances the body's need for movement and stretching, it also produces powerful feelings of well-being and happiness.

My interest in oriental medicine was so aroused that I also undertook to study Tui Na Chinese massage and acupuncture in China. After several visits to China, I subsequently returned to Thailand to study Thai massage at the sacred Wat Pho temple in Bangkok and the Old Medical Hospital in Chiang Mai. I also received private tuition from Chaiyuth Priyasith, one of Thailand's most respected masters.

In order to give others the opportunity to experience these ancient, yet thriving oriental therapies, I established the BODYHARMONICS® Centre in Cheltenham, England. Treatments and training in Thai bodywork and Indonesian traditional massage, Tui Na Chinese massage and acupuncture are provided there. Today all the members of my family share my passion for traditional oriental bodywork.

I believe that Thai traditional massage reaches those parts of the body and mind that other forms of massage fail to reach, and I hope that by reading this book you too will be motivated to try it and experience its unique benefits yourself.

M. B. Mercati

OPPOSITE: *These wonderfully ornate pagodas are characteristic of the Wat Pho, the temple where the author experienced her first traditional Thai massage. This manual will help you to discover healing benefits of Thai massage for yourself, your friends and family.*

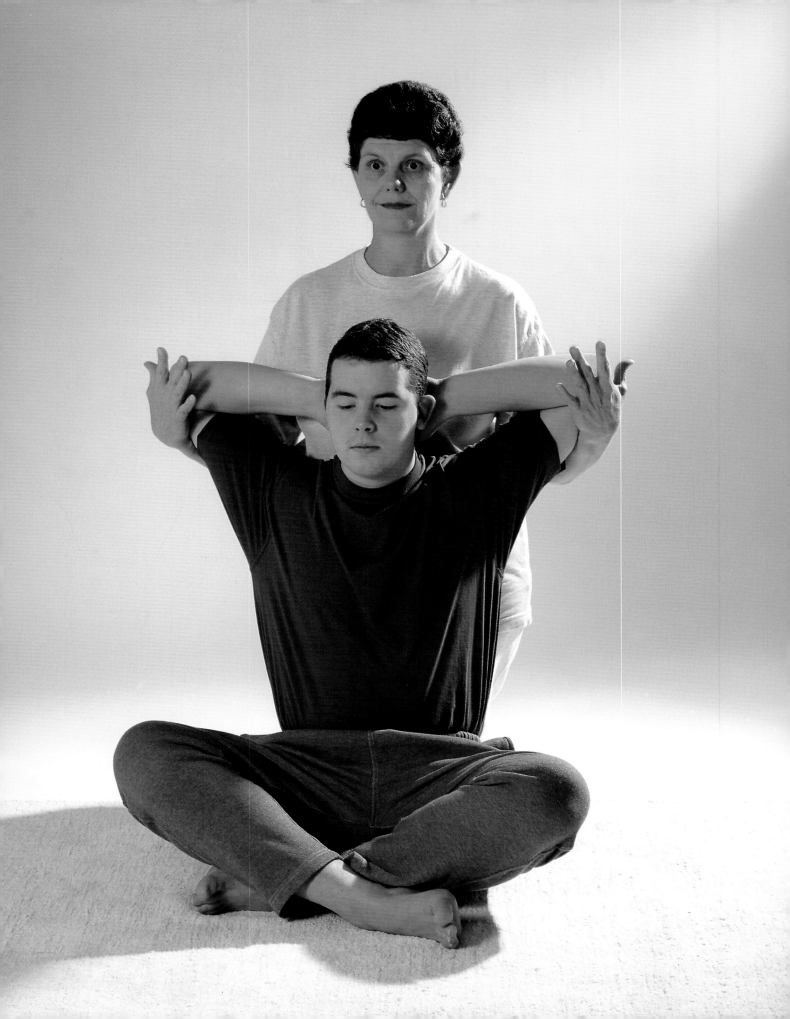

PART ONE
INTRODUCTION
นวดไทยโบราณ

Thai massage is one of the ancient healing arts of traditional Thai medicine, the others being herbal medicine and spiritual meditation. The term 'massage' conjures up images of something quite different from Thai massage, which even at its most basic, is a very complex sequence soft tissue pressing, stretching, twisting and joint manipulations. For this reason the author prefers to use the term 'Thai bodywork' rather than 'massage', which is used frequently throughout the book.

Thai bodywork has been in a process of constant evolution for over 1,000 years. It is not surprising, therefore, to find many subtle variations in the techniques used by different practitioners, and even greater differences are apparent between the styles of bodywork characteristic of the North and South of Thailand. The techniques presented by Maria Mercati in this book are essentially a 'pot pourri' of those taken from various regions of the country. Beginners will find them flowing and harmonious and very similar to what one could expect to receive at the hands of a Thai master.

ABOVE: *The Thai script means 'ancient massage'.*
OPPOSITE: *The author performs a Butterfly Shoulder Stretch on her son, Graham* (see page 131).

Traditional Thai Massage

Traditional Thai massage has been practised in more or less its present form for at least 1,000 years. It is a member of the whole family of Oriental bodywork, which is based on the intrinsic energy flow and energy balance theory of health and healing. Other members of this family include Tui Na Chinese massage and manipulation, Ayurvedic Indian massage and Shiatsu Japanese massage. Tui Na and Ayurvedic massage both date back over 4,000 years and it is in these systems that Thai massage has its roots. The Indian yogic influence is very obvious to both the observer and recipient of this unique form of massage. Less so, is the extremely disciplined manner in which the energy channels known as Sen (*see page 14*) are treated. In this respect, Thai bodywork more closely resembles Tui Na, the theory and practice of which was already documented some 2,300 years ago. The first ever recorded Western commentary regarding Thai medicine was made in 1690 by Simon de la Loubère, a French diplomat, who observed: 'When any person is sick at Siam he begins with causing his whole body to be moulded by one who is skilful herein, who gets upon the body of the sick person and tramples him under his feet.'

The role of Thai massage

Who needs traditional Thai massage and manipulation? You do, if your body is crying out: 'Touch me', 'Stretch me', 'Squeeze me', 'Hold me', 'Listen to me', 'Comfort me' or 'Heal me'. Such body cries often go unheard. This book will help you to discover how Thai bodywork can be the answer to your body's pleas and it could be the first important step that leads you to seek its unique benefits.

Modern lifestyles are often dominated by the desire to achieve independence and fulfilment through the use of machinery and new technology. We aim to make our lives easy and convenient and, with ever more leisure time, hope that we will be healthy, youthful and pain-free enough to enjoy life. There is a distinct trend towards self over-indulgence and this, unfortunately, goes hand in hand with increasing deprivation in areas such as regular exercise and interaction with others on a caring and compassionate level. This book is written in the firm belief that Thai bodywork involves just such an interaction, enabling you to share with another person in a mutual 'un-Thai-ing' of physical and emotional knots. Interaction through physical contact has been fundamental to most Eastern cultures for thousands of years, yet the practice still remains quite foreign to most Westerners.

At this point, it must be emphasized that traditional Thai massage is not the same thing as the media-sensationalized activities that take place in massage parlours throughout the tourist centres of Thailand. It is not about sexual gratification but about wholeness, balance, health and happiness. Thai massage means togetherness at a physical level which is quite outside the sexual but, for all of us, this is one of the vital components of a happy, balanced life that is so often lacking in this modern world.

The origins of traditional Thai massage

Like the origins of the Thai people themselves, the history of traditional Thai massage is obscure. Thailand was at the crossroads of the ancient migration routes which saw many waves of different civilizations and cultures passing through. The combination of Thailand's close proximity to China and its position on one of the main trade routes from India has resulted in many interesting cultural and religious influences, particularly Buddhism, being brought to bear on the early inhabitants of this area.

Folk tradition credits Jivaka Kumar Bhaccha, also known as Shiuago Komparaj, with being the founder of Thai massage. A friend and

OPPOSITE: *A monk, in traditional orange robes, walks across the courtyard in front of the Wat Pho temple, the national centre for the teaching and preservation of traditional Thai medicine.*

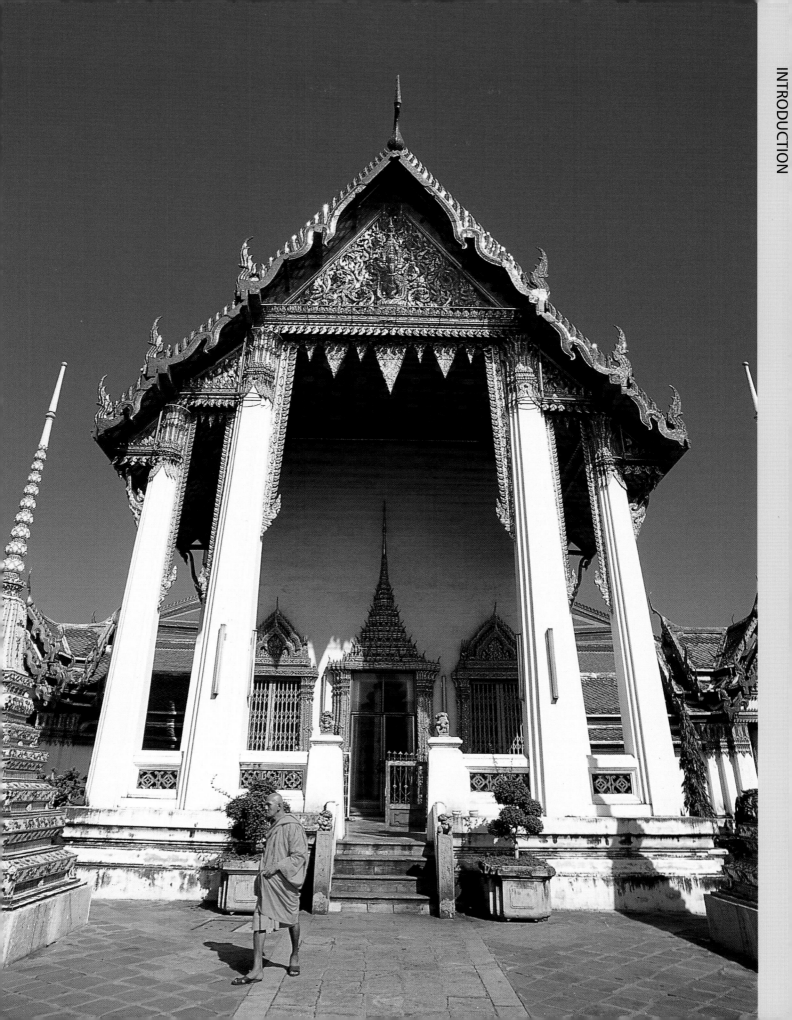

physician to the Buddha some 2,500 years ago, he is still revered as the 'Father of Thai medicine'. None of the information regarding massage procedures was written down and it was passed on from generation to generation by word of mouth. Medical texts that included detailed descriptions of Thai massage, as it was then practised, were eventually recorded in the Pali language on palm leaves. These were venerated as religious texts and held in safe keeping in the old capital city of Ayutthia. During the eighteenth century Ayulthia was overrun by Burmese invaders and many of the precious texts were destroyed. In 1832 King Rama III had all the surviving texts carved in stone as descriptive epigraphs at Wat Pho, the largest temple in Bangkok.

Wat Pho temple

'Wats' are temples or monasteries. Besides being focal points for the practice of Buddhism, the Wats have always provided for the health needs of the people. The Wat Pho is the most famous of them. It dates back to the sixteenth century and houses the famous reclining Buddha, which is 46 metres (150 feet) long and 15 metres (49 feet) high, together with the largest collection of Buddha images in Thailand. There are sixty carved epigraphs that describe the Sen channels and embody all the information from the Pali texts that still survived during the reign of King Rama III. Outside the temple are a collection of stone statues that show various of the classical Thai massage techniques.

Wat Pho is the national centre for the teaching and preservation of traditional Thai medicine. Most Thais are Buddhists and even today they are devoted to Buddha's teachings of non-violence, loving kindness and compassion. Monks are still supported by gifts of food from the people and making regular offerings at the temples is regarded as virtuous. The monarchy is based on Buddhist teachings and has enormous popular support. The present king, Bhumibol Adulyadej, is the ninth monarch in direct succession.

With its origins firmly rooted in Buddhist philosophy, it is not surprising that, for much of its history, traditional Thai massage has been regarded as a religious rite. Until quite recently Thai massage was only officially practised by monks which, of course, precluded women as potential recipients. Various forms of folk massage were, and still are, practised within families where family members massaged one another.

The Sen lines

In Thai medical theory the body's vital life energy flows along channels called Sen. This energy powers all the physical, mental and emotional processes which will only function normally when energy supply matches demand. The Chinese call this energy 'Qi' and the Indians call it 'Prana'. Any imbalance or blockage in the distribution of this energy can cause pain and disease. When the system is working well and energy distribution is balanced, you feel happy, relaxed, energetic and free from stiffness and pain.

Thai massage focuses on the main Sen channels. The careful application of pressure along these channels helps to release any energy blockages and stagnation. Pressing and stretching muscles makes them more receptive to this flow. In Part Two of this book each lesson begins with a diagram of the Sen channels to guide your pressing as you then massage the relevant section of the body. In addition to this, dots and arrows have been superimposed over the colour photographs of many of the techniques so that you can see clearly the direction, and the full range of movement involved in all the manipulations.

What Thai bodywork can do for you

Yoga is generally accepted as being an effective way of remaining healthy and flexible. However, receiving Thai bodywork is the ultimate lazy and simple way of obtaining all the benefits of yoga and more – without having to do it yourself. And when it is your turn to give your partner a massage, you will also feel the benefits of being the giver.

This book will guide you towards mastering a comprehensive range of Thai massage and manipulation techniques, and presents you

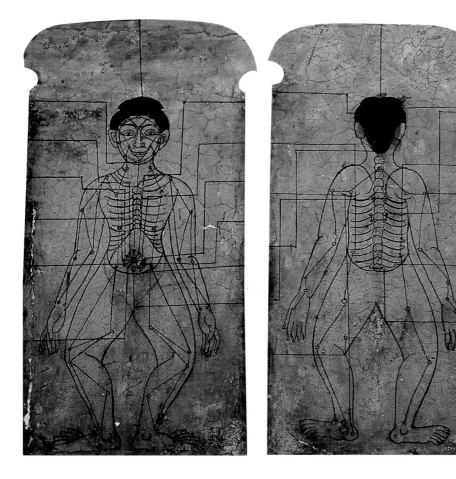

LEFT: *These are two of the descriptive epigraphs that were etched in stone by order of King Rama III. The complete series can be seen at Wat Pho and represents all the surviving ancient texts on Thai traditional massage.*

with a flowing sequence that can be used to maintain the body in a youthful condition. The techniques can also be used as a healing treatment for chronic pain *(see Part Three)*.

Stiffness and loss of flexibility are regarded as the inevitable result of the ageing process in the Western world. How you feel – physically, mentally and emotionally – is more important than your mere physical age. Thai bodywork is unique in its ability to preserve youthfulness.

The secret of Thai bodywork

What is the secret of Thai bodywork? The answer is that it enables you to press your muscles and to balance energy levels. This is what affects flexibility and equalizes the effects of muscles on both sides of the body. The amount of movement a muscle can produce at a joint is determined by the difference between its length when relaxed and when fully contracted. When muscles are tense, they become shorter, even when you are not consciously contracting them. This can happen through overworking them, by not using them

enough or it could be due to emotional tension. Whatever the cause may be, the end result is progressively more restricted movement and the onset of stiffness, aches and pains which are all characteristic of the ageing process.

Muscles that shorten and become tense can create uneven forces on the spine – that all-important container of the spinal cord. This, in turn, creates the back pain, neck pain and headaches that can so easily become a regular feature of daily life. With its unique ability to stretch all the most important muscles in the body systematically, Thai manipulations enable you to achieve effects which are unlike those of any other bodywork.

Thai bodywork should not be regarded as a mere physical experience. Indeed, if that is all it turns out to be, then it has largely failed to achieve its real potential. The giving and receiving of Thai bodywork is an ideal way of providing for the subtle, yet powerful interchange of intrinsic energy between two individuals. It is always a *two-way* process, and achievement depends on the caring and

13

compassionate way in which it is given. Even in this day and age, Thai bodywork is a vital necessity for everyday life because it underpins health and well-being. It is the perfect vehicle for two people to come together with a view to attaining this mutual balancing of energy and life-force. Thai bodywork embodies all the harmony and rhythm often lacking in our lives.

Thai bodywork in practice

The many techniques used in Thai bodywork are all designed to facilitate and stimulate the flow of intrinsic energies and to release blockages that would otherwise preclude the attainment of balance that is essential for maintaining a healthy, pain-free body. In this context, 'healthy' and 'pain-free' refer not only to the purely physical but also to the mental, emotional and spiritual aspects of one's being.

In this book you will find over 150 different techniques that can be used in a massage. Feet, palms, thumbs, elbows and knees are all used to apply deep pressure along the Sen. Other, quite different techniques, are used to apply twists and stretches, and these resemble a kind of applied yoga. At all times the pace is measured and unhurried. When moving from one technique to the next, the movement should be rhythmical, flowing, harmonious and smooth.

Thai bodywork starts in the supine position – lying on the back – and then each side is worked. This is followed by the prone position – lying face downwards – and the sequence finishes in the sitting position. This routine always begins with the feet, which are subjected to a variety of presses, stretches and flexion that would even surprise a reflexologist! The legs are systematically positioned through a range of postures that present the energy channels to their best advantage.

However, it is for its manipulations that Thai bodywork is renowned. These are designed to stretch every accessible muscle *just a little more* than it would normally be stretched under the action of strongly contracting antagonistic muscles. In the process, all the principal joints are likewise moved *just a little*

more than when they are operating under their own muscle power.

Touch me, stretch me

Touch is one of the greatest medicines. It soothes, releases and comforts. Our wholeness is nourished by frequent and regular doses of this all-pervading medicine.

In this context, wholeness includes spiritual and emotional aspects as well as the more easily observed physical ones. When looked at with a knowledge of Western medicine, it is easy to see how massage and manipulation can stimulate the flow of blood and lymph (tissue fluid), warm the tissues, improve flexibility and ease pain, all of which are essentially physical.

Such is the power of touch that it also reaches far into the hidden recesses of our being. It has been shown that touch can result in the release of chemical substances within the nervous system called endorphins, which counteract pain and produce a powerful feeling of well-being.

Thai bodywork involves different forms of touch – pressing, stretching and twisting – which have been honed to perfection over the ages. Those who receive Thai bodywork regularly will experience feelings of relaxation, peace of mind, happiness, flexibility and youthfulness.

Heal me

The word 'heal' suggests ill health or disease, but its meaning in the context in which it is used here requires a much wider definition of health than is commonly recognized. Health is not just physical well-being or general lack of disease; it is a statement regarding the balance that exists between all those factors which contribute to our sense of 'wholeness', both internal and external. Whilst it would be difficult to give any accurate, all-embracing definition of what constitutes health, it is characterized by feelings of vitality, flexibility, freedom from pain, contentment and a sense of wholeness.

The healthy person has, above all else, a balance in his or her life. One of the adverse spin-offs from life in the fast lane is a disturbance of this balance and when this happens, one has to have time and space in which to restore that elusive equilibrium. Sharing Thai bodywork with a partner or receiving it from a qualified practitioner is certainly one of the most effective means of doing this.

Stay young, stay healthy

Pain is the biggest single obstacle to happiness and pain of any kind, at any level, is a reflection of imbalance. This results from too much of some things and not enough of others. The body will experience pain if, for example, it has too much rich food or too much violent exercise. But pains of no less a magnitude will be experienced if insufficient food is eaten and no exercise is taken. Pain will also be experienced when the desires of the mind remain unfulfilled but equally intense pain will be felt when desire is so restricted that there is no driving force for any progress.

The quest for health should be regarded as the search for balance in every facet of our lives. Rest and relaxation are wonderful ways of calming the mind and body to help this balancing process which we commonly call 'healing' and there are many things that we can do in our daily lives which can help to make it happen. Receiving Thai bodywork is one of them. Simultaneously, Thai bodywork can give a sublimely rhythmical workout that perfectly balances the body's need for movement and stretching, whilst it also provides a relaxed state in which excessive worry and desire seem to evaporate away.

'The Four Divine States of Consciousness'

As I have mentioned earlier, traditional Thai massage was originally practised in Buddhist temples because of its religious significance. It was regarded as one of the many ways of working towards the 'Four Divine States of Consciousness' and for Buddhists these are a necessary prerequisite for complete happiness. The qualities embodied in these states are:

- METTA: *The desire to make others happy and the ability to show loving kindness*
- KARUNA: *Compassion for all who suffer and a desire to ease their sufferings*
- MUDITA: *Rejoicing with those who have good fortune and never feeling envy*
- UPEKKHA: *Regarding one's fellows without prejudice or preference.*

From the Buddhist viewpoint, the giver of massage should be motivated only by the desire to bestow loving kindness with total concern for the recipient's physical and emotional pains and feelings. Massage given with these motives foremost is a healing experience for the giver as well as the receiver, and intrinsic life energy will flow between the two.

Thai bodywork treatment

In order to give and to receive Thai bodywork, you will need a partner – your spouse, friend or perhaps a member of your family. It is most important that you should avoid working with anyone who is much heavier than yourself, particularly when carrying out exercises that may involve heavy lifting or standing on your partner. Thai bodywork is, above all else, an intimate and warm experience and it should be carried out in an environment which promotes these features. A warm, well-ventilated room with diffused or subdued lighting is most conducive to the meditative state of the giver and the relaxation of the receiver. It is important that there should be no disturbances or excessive noise, although some people may prefer to have gentle background music played throughout the massage. As the bodywork is carried out on the floor, a soft but supportive mat or blanket should be used, together with a thin pillow to support the receiver's head. Adequate space should be provided to enable the giver to move comfortably around the receiver.

Thai massage is applied to the clothed body but it is usual for the receiver to be barefoot. It is helpful if clothing takes the form of a thin, natural-fibre track suit or similar type of loose garment, and this is ideal wear for the giver who is also barefoot.

Before giving a massage to someone for the first time it is most important that you

15

check their medical history and discuss any present health problems with them before commencing *(see page 17)*. Immediately before any physical contact is made, you should take a moment to clear your mind of all extraneous thoughts so as to be totally centred on your partner's needs and to be able to attend to them in a calm and empathetic state. A few slow, deep breaths with controlled exhalation will help this relaxing process.

Before starting a massage, a Thai practitioner says a prayer to the Father of Medicine asking for guidance and help in relieving the physical and emotional pain in the patient. You too can say a prayer if you wish.

Throughout the massage your partner should breathe normally except when receiving the 'Cobras' *(see pages 120-123)* and Lifting Spinal Twist *(see page 109)*. Breathing in deeply before the lifts commence and breathing out as the lifts take place encourages energy flow to the internal organs. As with all forms of massage, pace, rhythm and pressure must be carefully controlled and, above all else, there must be a sense of continuous flow, not only from technique to technique but also of energies within the partnership between giver and receiver. In this book wherever possible the first word used in the headings for the exercises refers to the action of the giver or, where appropriate, the body part used by the giver.

The duration of a massage

A Thai massage can take from two to two-and-a-half hours to complete but this does not preclude the possibility of effective massage when there is less time. It is much better to restrict massage to those regions of the body that can be adequately treated in the time available than to speed up and attempt to do a whole body massage in a much shorter time. A selection of short programmes to treat specific conditions is listed in Part Three. In addition, a basic routine for the beginner is given at the end of the book *(see page 141)*. If you are new to bodywork do not attempt the more advanced manipulations until you are able to do the basic routine smoothly and effectively.

Beware of over-stretching

Over-stretching can cause injury. After just a short experience of giving massage it soon becomes very apparent that every individual has a different pain threshold, sensitivity and overall flexibility. When applied to some people, deep pressure produces little more than a mild sensation, whereas for others mild pressure can – at times – be quite excruciating. Flexibility and tolerance of stretching show the same variability. It is most important that one learns to recognize quickly to what degree pressure and stretching can be used. Pressing can cause pain if applied too vigorously. Always start with light pressure and increase very slowly. Use visual clues from your partner to guide you as to the maximum pressure to use.

It is always important to get verbal confirmation from your partner that the stretches are not excessive. Age is no indication of suppleness and pain threshold. Some very young people can be stiff whereas others in their seventies who have cared for their bodies can demonstrate a remarkable flexibility.

Caring for yourself

Good balance and posture are of vital significance for the giver of Thai bodywork as muscular strain can easily be sustained if unnatural and stressful positions are adopted. Leaning in with the full body weight is a far more effective way of applying pressure and performing some of the extensive stretching movements than trying to achieve these with only the muscular power of the arms and shoulders. The giver should feel as comfortable as the receiver since any discomfort will interrupt concentration and destroy the harmony of movement that is so characteristic of good Thai bodywork.

Rhythm and movement: a pure synthesis

The words 'flowing' and 'rhythmic' exactly describe the essence of Thai bodywork with its sequence of unhurried presses, stretches and twists. For the beginner, the vast number, variety and the subtlety of techniques used may be somewhat bewildering. At all times, the position and movements of the giver in relation to the receiver are every bit as important as the way in which the techniques are applied. Nuances of tempo and pressure seem endless and one technique dissolves into another with total smoothness and harmony. Form seems as important as movement. The symmetries and shapes developed and sustained are as dramatic as the way in which they evaporate away. There is never a suggestion of haste, and to the receiver time seems almost to stand still.

Thai bodywork is a fusion of techniques, each of them with its own specific effect. Some techniques apply pressure to the Sen channels *(see page 14)* while others produce the wonderful twists and stretches that often resemble applied yoga. Pressing is the means of stimulating movement of energy in the Sen channels and manipulations stretch muscles. Feet, palms, thumbs, elbows and knees are the tools of the Thai therapist. The unhurried pace and smooth flow that characterize this form of bodywork detracts from the very deep pressure and powerful stretches that are used. Thai bodywork is like a beautifully choreographed duet: the basic theme is repeated over and over again, but with subtle variations for each body part that is treated.

CONTRA-INDICATIONS TO THAI MASSAGE

A few words of caution must be stated. All those incredible shapes and flowing movements that constitute the manipulative side of Thai massage can be potentially damaging to both giver and receiver. To give a massage of this kind, at even a very modest level, requires great skill, strength and poise which can only be acquired with correct training. Even a fit young person can be hurt when subjected to stretches and twists that are incorrectly applied or simply overdone. In addition, there are the usual contra-indications to the use of Thai massage which are essentially those that would apply to any form of massotherapy:

WHEN NOT TO USE THAI BODYWORK

- *Do not massage anyone with a serious heart condition, high blood pressure or cancer.*
- *Thai massage is unsuitable for those who sufferer from brittle bones (osteoporosis).*
- *Never massage anyone who has an artificial joint, such as a hip or knee replacement.*
- *Those suffering from skin conditions such as eczema, psoriasis or shingles should not receive massage on the affected areas.*
- *Many of the exercises in this book are unsuitable for pregnant women and Thai massage is* **not** *recommended during pregnancy.*
- *Varicose veins should not be deeply massaged.*
- *If the receiver has any condition that raises doubts in the mind of the giver as to the suitability of this type of massage it is always best to err on the side of caution and to refer this person to his or her doctor, who may be able to determine whether massage is contra-indicated.*

CHAPTER 1

THE MUSCLES
TARGETS FOR THE THAI THERAPIST

Ageing is often more to do with how we feel than with the passage of time. Decreasing flexibility, stiffness, tension, aches and pains all contribute to the feeling of getting old. Most chronic pain – even headaches – is associated with the musculo-skeletal system and originates from muscles which remain contracted (stay shortened) even in their 'relaxed' state. Muscles are the anatomical targets of the Thai masseur.

Skeletal muscle is contractile tissue. It provides the force (effort) for all voluntary movement. Muscles are attached to bone (or sometimes connective tissue or cartilage) by means of tendons. These are flexible and enormously strong, inelastic structures that arise from the connective tissue that covers the muscles. At their outer ends, tendons fuse with connective tissue that covers the bone or cartilage. Whenever a muscle contracts, it shortens and this creates a pull that is transmitted through the tendons to bring about movement.

The superficial muscles of the body

In the living body, the superficial muscles cover layers of deep muscles which, in turn, may cover even deeper muscles. Seen here, the relationship between the body's natural curves and the superficial muscles beneath the skin and subcutaneous fat is clear. Some deep muscles (shaded orange) can be glimpsed beneath the superficial muscles.

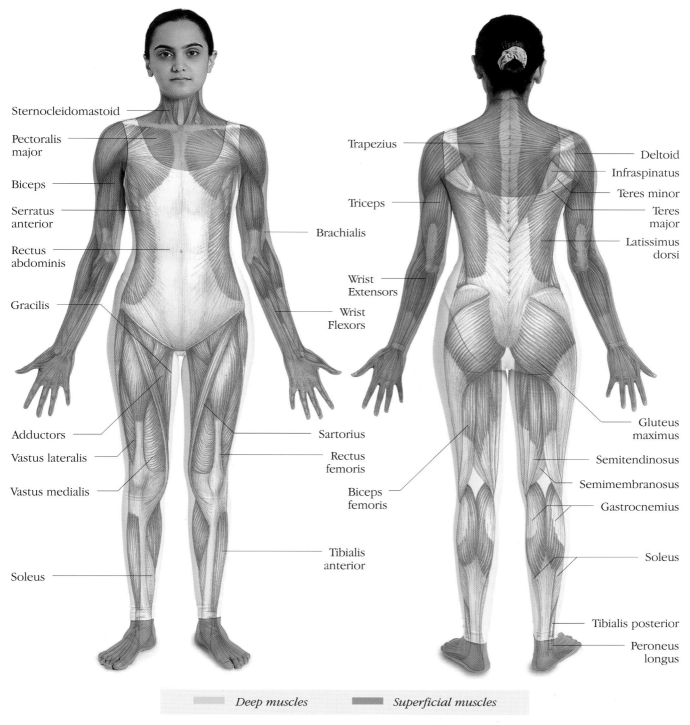

Sternocleidomastoid

Pectoralis major

Biceps

Serratus anterior

Rectus abdominis

Gracilis

Adductors

Vastus lateralis

Vastus medialis

Soleus

Trapezius

Triceps

Brachialis

Wrist Extensors

Wrist Flexors

Sartorius

Rectus femoris

Biceps femoris

Tibialis anterior

Deltoid

Infraspinatus

Teres minor

Teres major

Latissimus dorsi

Gluteus maximus

Semitendinosus

Semimembranosus

Gastrocnemius

Soleus

Tibialis posterior

Peroneus longus

Deep muscles   *Superficial muscles*

How Muscles Work

Muscles act on the bones, and these form a very complex system of levers. A muscle is usually attached by its tendons to the bones positioned on either side of a joint. Whenever the muscle contracts, the joint acts like a pivot and movement is created between the bones.

Muscle cannot work by itself; it depends upon many other tissues, such as myofascia. This not only provides the outer covering for the muscle but also penetrates deeply within the muscle, binding together bundles of muscle fibres and carrying nerves and blood capillaries deep into the muscle tissue. Indeed, all the organs of the body depend upon connective tissue for support and to bind their various components together. It is connective tissue that forms the supporting framework for the dense network of blood capillaries, nerves and lymph vessels that are essential components of the muscular system. It also provides the ultra-smooth surfaces that enable each muscle to move against its neighbours with almost no friction. Painful adhesions occur when this property of the connective tissue is disturbed.

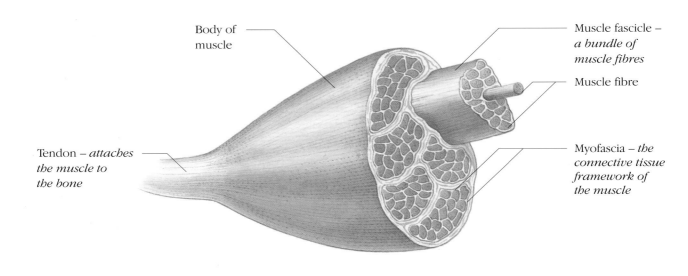

Body of muscle

Muscle fascicle – *a bundle of muscle fibres*

Muscle fibre

Tendon – *attaches the muscle to the bone*

Myofascia – *the connective tissue framework of the muscle*

Diagram of muscle tissue (enlarged)
This sectioned muscle shows the arrangement of the tissues that provide for its supporting framework and its contractile ability.

The Central Nervous System
The brain and spinal cord make up the *central nervous system (CNS)* which is the controlling computer for all body parts, both involuntary (such as breathing) and voluntary, such as the skeletal muscles. Muscles are linked to the central nervous system by two kinds of nerves:

• *Motor nerves:* these carry nerve impulses from the CNS to make the muscles contract.

• *Sensory nerves:* these carry nerve impulses from sense organs in the muscles to the CNS.

The sense organs in muscles are called *spindle organs* because of their shape. They provide constant information about the state of muscle contraction and any change in it. The tendons also contain sense organs which tell the brain how much pull they are being subjected to as the muscles contract.

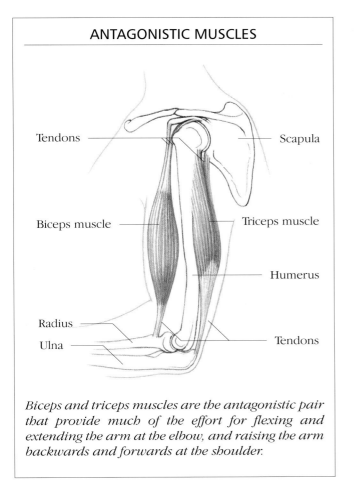

ANTAGONISTIC MUSCLES

Tendons

Scapula

Biceps muscle

Triceps muscle

Humerus

Radius

Ulna

Tendons

Biceps and triceps muscles are the antagonistic pair that provide much of the effort for flexing and extending the arm at the elbow, and raising the arm backwards and forwards at the shoulder.

What is a muscle?

A muscle is a bundle of vast numbers of muscle fibres, all arranged lengthwise and parallel with one another. Muscle fibres are the basic contractile elements within muscles. All muscle fibres have the ability to contract and thus shorten. They contract in an 'all-or-nothing' way and it is not possible for a muscle fibre to contract just a little. Full contraction or no contraction are the only two possibilities.

Different muscle fibres respond in different ways to the impulses that arrive through motor nerves. Some have what is called low threshold response. This means that they contract under very low frequency of motor-nerve stimulation. Others are far less sensitive and need much higher frequency stimulation. These are said to have a high threshold. Within the same muscle there are muscle fibres with differing thresholds, to cover the complete spectrum, from low to high. The different response

thresholds of the individual muscle fibres allow the muscle to contract *smoothly* and *progressively* as more of them come into action as motor-nerve stimulation increases.

Functional muscle groups

Smooth, variable, co-ordinated movement results from muscles functioning in groups. A group that flexes a joint, for example, interacts with and opposes the action of one that extends it. Two such groups of muscles are said to be *antagonistic*. Biceps and triceps are the main muscles from the antagonistic groups that flex and extend the elbow. Other major functional groups are the quadriceps muscles, which extend the knee and flex the thigh, and the hamstring muscles, which flex the knee and extend the thigh. Each of the four quadriceps and three hamstring muscles works slightly differently from the others to include a degree of rotation in either direction.

Muscles at rest

Muscles can only contract, they cannot actively stretch. When a muscle stops contracting it depends on its antagonists to stretch it back to its normal relaxed length when they contract. Even an apparently relaxed muscle has a small proportion of its fibres in a contracted state. These give a muscle its *tone*. Muscle tone depends on a constant, low-frequency motor-nerve stimulation that originates in the brain. It is just enough to keep the lowest-threshold fibres contracted. Any disturbance of normal tone can seriously affect muscle function. Deficient tone makes the muscle limp and flaccid so that part of its potential contraction is used to 'take up the slack' instead of producing movement. Too much tone deceives the brain into thinking that the muscle is contracting, and so inhibits some of the contractile ability of the antagonists, which gradually weaken as a result.

The sheer complexity of muscle interaction is reflected in Thai bodywork, which treats every muscle from every angle.

The Therapeutic Effects of Thai Bodywork

Pressing and stretching are where Thai bodywork excels. At this point it is appropriate to look at what happens to our muscles and how pressing and stretching can help them. One of the most common muscle problems is a gradual shortening of the relaxed muscle length. This has many causes. Those who do too much heavy, repetitive manual work or weight training in the gym can develop muscles with higher than normal tone. This is due to increased numbers of muscle fibres remaining contracted, even when the muscle is in its 'relaxed' state. Other factors such as injury, poor posture and emotional stress can also cause this to happen.

The most immediate effect of muscle shortening is reduced movement at the joint where the muscle works. This is because the difference between the relaxed length and the contracted length of the muscle is less than it should be. Unfortunately, it is this difference that determines how much movement the muscle can produce, so stiffness and reduced joint mobility is the result of muscle shortening.

Other unpleasant conditions can also prevail. When a muscle becomes tense and shortened, its spindle organs send impulses to the brain which tell it that the muscle is in a state of contraction. The brain now responds by reducing motor stimulation to its antagonistic muscle. This muscle now loses tone and, if the condition persists, it will gradually weaken. Soon it will not even match the strength of its antagonist, which will shorten still further since it will not be pulled hard enough to stretch it. A state of imbalance quickly results which, in some cases, can produce postural problems leading to chronic pain.

This is not yet the end of the story! The myofascia has large areas between its cells which contain fibres. Some of these are elastic; some are not. The non-elastic ones serve to strengthen the tissue. As a muscle shortens, the myofascia contracts and shortens with it. Gradually it loses some of its elasticity, if it is not repeatedly stretched to what should be the correct relaxed length of the muscle. Elastic fibres become replaced by the non-elastic kind and the tissue becomes slightly wrinkled. Movement of the neighbouring tissues becomes less smooth and this can cause discomfort which can also lead to abnormal use of the affected parts. As the myofascia shrinks due to lack of stretching, it thickens and becomes fibrotic, impeding normal muscle stretching during relaxation and further reducing movement and joint mobility. All these interrelated effects mean pain, stiffness, lowered resistance to joint injury and reduced performance on the sports field.

The benefits of pressing and stretching

The deep presses of Thai bodywork squash the muscles, stretching the myofascia sideways. This helps to break down fibrotic tissue and stimulates the production of elastic fibres. Blood flow through the myofascial capillaries is enhanced and energy flow through the Sen is improved. These changes help to alleviate pain and make all the tissues amenable to the effects of stretching that are to follow.

The large-scale, sustained stretches that characterize Thai manipulations are applied in a myriad different directions. The practitioner constantly changes the angle of approach by altering the relative positions of different parts of the body. Stretching of muscles – even those that are abnormally shortened – takes them just beyond what their normal relaxed length would be. Muscle spindle organs respond to this by 'telling' the brain that the muscle is relaxed, inhibitory nerve impulses to the antagonistic muscles stop and they soon regain normal tone. Regular Thai bodywork stretches comprehensively restore balance within and between functional groups of muscles to ease pain, increase flexibility and improve posture.

Improving and maintaining flexibility

The overall flexibility of the body's movable joints starts to diminish from the early twenties unless positive steps are taken to work them

SHORTENED MUSCLES

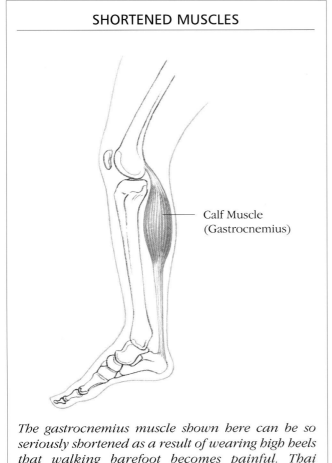

Calf Muscle
(Gastrocnemius)

The gastrocnemius muscle shown here can be so seriously shortened as a result of wearing high heels that walking barefoot becomes painful. Thai massage easily corrects this condition.

through a wide range of movements at regular intervals. The practice of yoga could achieve this but reaching an adequate level of expertise requires much application and discipline. Thai massage, on the other hand, requires nothing more than placing your body in the hands of an expert practitioner. After a session lasting around two to two-and-a-half hours your muscles and joints will have received an intensive workout, the thoroughness of which you could never hope to equal by yourself. The improvement in your flexibility will be noticeable immediately. This is because Thai bodywork always stretches muscles and manipulates joints just a little further than you would be capable of when unaided.

The treatment of many conditions

Though unsuitable for people with serious health problems and those who have had replacement surgery, for others Thai bodywork can seem like a miracle in the way it treats those conditions that result from physical and emotional stress. Repetitive strain injuries, wear and tear and sports injuries are the commonest results of physical stress. The signals that warn you of its effects vary from stiffness, weakness and pain to serious loss of performance. The indicators of emotional stress are vastly more complex. They can be purely emotional, such as worry, anxiety and anger, or behavioural, as with over-eating and alcohol, tobacco and drug abuse. Inability to relax, disrupted sleep patterns and general irritability are also observed. Eventually, emotional stress manifests itself through a range of physical symptoms that include headaches, indigestion, constipation, back pains and skin conditions.

Enhancing sports performance

A flexible body is one of the keys to fitness and performance. The other is a musculature with total balance between antagonistic groups, with every individual muscle able to assume its normal relaxed length when not contracting. This is probably a combination that even the most highly trained athletes fail to achieve. Including Thai bodywork as part of their training regime can help all sportsmen and women towards this ideal condition. It will enable them to undertake more intensive training with a significantly reduced risk of injury, and this will result in an ability to sustain even higher levels of performance safely .

Treating sports injuries

Most sports injuries involve damage to muscle fibres, myofascia or tendons and they are commonly caused by overuse of muscles that are not functionally balanced with other muscles in their group and with their antagonists. A healthy, normal muscle has an amazing capacity to perform repetitively without injury. Thai bodywork received regularly provides maintenance that the muscles need. When injury does occur, its controlled stretches and manipulations have an unrivalled ability to speed healing and restore normal pain-free function.

❧ The Muscles ❧

Head and Neck

MUSCLE	REGION LESSON	ATTACHMENTS (origin and insertion)	MUSCLE ACTION	KEY THAI MANIPULATIONS ACTING ON THE MUSCLE
Erector spinae (Sacrospinalis) (see also page 27)	Head and neck Lessons 3, 5 & 8	O: Lower-neck (cervical) vertebrae, upper-back (thoracic) vertebrae I: Upper cervical vertebrae, base of skull and ribs	(Both sides) Holds neck erect and bends it backwards. (One side) Flexes head and neck sideways	• Bow & Arrow Spinal Twist *(see page 78)* • Pulling the Turned Head *(see page 96)* • Interlocked Hand/Neck Press *(see page 126)* • Seated Lateral Arm Lever *(see page 129)* • Butterfly Shoulder Stretch *(see page 131)* • Butterfly Manipulation *(see page 131)*
Sternocleido-mastoid	Head and neck Lessons 5 & 8	O: Mastoid bone behind ear I: Top of breast bone (sternum), collar bone (clavicle)	(Both sides) Tilts head forwards (One side) Turns head towards shoulder on that side	• Pulling the Turned Head *(see page 96)* • Stretching the Neck & Shoulders *(see page 126)* • Seated Lateral Arm Lever *(see page 129)*

Trapezius

Sternocleidomastoid
Levator scapulae
Rhomboideus minor
Deltoid
Infraspinatus
Teres major
Serratus anterior
Erector spinae

MUSCLE	REGION LESSON	ATTACHMENTS (origin and insertion)	MUSCLE ACTION	KEY THAI MANIPULATIONS ACTING ON THE MUSCLE
Levator scapulae	Head and neck Lessons 3, 5 & 8	O: First four cervical vertebrae I: Top inner angle of the shoulder blade (scapula)	Raises shoulder blade and pulls it towards spine	• Bow & Arrow Spinal Twist *(see page 78)* • Pulling the Turned Head *(see page 96)* • Interlocked Hand/Neck Press *(see page 126)* • Seated Lateral Arm Lever *(see page 129)*

Head and Neck continued

MUSCLE	REGION LESSON	ATTACHMENTS *(origin and insertion)*	MUSCLE ACTION	KEY THAI MANIPULATIONS ACTING ON THE MUSCLE
Trapezius	Head and neck Lessons 3, 5, 7 & 8	O: Base of skull (occiput), cervical vertebrae two to six via the nuchal ligament, and the last cervical and all thoracic vertebrae I: Outer end of collarbone (clavicle), spine of shoulder blade (scapula)	Rotates and raises shoulder blades. (One side) Flexes and rotates neck	• Bow & Arrow Spinal Twist *(see page 78)* • Lifting Head to Straight Knees *(see page 85)* • Lifting Head to Crossed Knees *(see page 85)* • Foot to Armpit Stretch *(see page 92)* • Pulling the Arms *(see page 95)* • Pulling the Turned Head *(see page 96)* • Rotating the Shoulder *(see page 102)* • Lifting Spinal Twist *(see page 109)* • Standing Cobra *(see page 121)* • Seated Lateral Arm Lever *(see page 129)*

Shoulders

MUSCLE	REGION LESSON	ATTACHMENTS *(origin and insertion)*	MUSCLE ACTION	KEY THAI MANIPULATIONS ACTING ON THE MUSCLE
Teres minor	Shoulder Lessons 3, 5 & 8	O: Outer margin of shoulder blade (scapula) I: Back of the head of humerus	Rotates arm outwards	• Lifting Head to Straight Knees *(see page 85)* • Lifting Head to Crossed Knees *(see page 85)* • Pulling the Arms *(see page 95)* • Backward Arm Lever *(see page 127)* • Elbow Pivot Lever *(see page 128)* • Stretching the Arm in the Triangle Position *(see page 128)* • Seated Lateral Arm Lever *(see page 129)* • Butterfly Shoulder Stretch *(see page 131)*
Teres major	Shoulder Lessons 3, 6 & 8	O: Lower half of outer margin of of shoulder blade (scapula) I: Inside margin on upper humerus	Extends arm backwards and rotates it inwards	• Lifting Head to Straight Knees *(see page 85)* • Lifting Head to Crossed Knees *(see page 85)* • Pulling the Arm in the Side Position *(see page 104)* • Stretching the Arm in the Triangle Position *(see page 105)* • Backward Arm Lever *(see page 127)* • Elbow Pivot Lever *(see page 128)* • Seated Lateral Arm Lever *(see page 129)* • Butterfly Shoulder Stretch *(see page 131)*
Supraspinatus	Shoulder Lessons 5, 6, 7 & 8	O: Shoulder blade above the spine (scapula) I: Outer margin on top of humerus	Raises arm (abducts)	• Foot to Armpit Stretch *(see page 92)* • Pulling Spinal Twist *(see page 109)* • Kneeling Cushion, Sitting Stool, Standing & Intimate Cobra *(see pages 118–119, 120, 121 & 123)* • Elbow Pivot Lever *(see page 128)* • Butterfly Shoulder Stretch *(see page 131)*
Infraspinatus	Shoulder Lessons 5, 6, 7 & 8	O: Inner shoulder blade I: Back of head of humerus	Rotates arm outwards	*As for supraspinatus* • Rotating the Shoulder *(see page 102)* • Lifting Spinal Twist *(see page 109)*
Subscapularis	Shoulder Lessons 3, 5, 6 & 8	O: Front of shoulder blade (scapula) I: Inner surface of upper humerus	Pulls arm downwards, rotates arm towards chest	*As for teres minor* • Lifting Spinal Twist *(see page 109)*

MUSCLE	REGION LESSON	ATTACHMENTS (origin and insertion)	MUSCLE ACTION	KEY THAI MANIPULATIONS ACTING ON THE MUSCLE
Deltoid	Shoulder Lessons 5, 6, 7 & 8	O: Collar bone and outer shoulder blade I: Humerus	Raises (abducts) arm	**As for supraspinatus** (see page 25)
Serratus anterior	Shoulder Lessons 7 & 8	O: Ribs 1-9 I: Inner margin of shoulder blade (scapula)	Antagonistic to rhomboideus muscles, helps to stabilize shoulder blade	• Kneeling Cushion, Sitting Stool and Standing Cobra (see pages 118–119, 120 & 121) • Feet to Back Stretch (see page 132)

Chest and Abdominal Muscles

MUSCLE	REGION LESSON	ATTACHMENTS (origin and insertion)	MUSCLE ACTION	KEY THAI MANIPULATIONS ACTING ON THE MUSCLE
Pectoralis major	Chest Lessons 5, 6, 7 & 8	O: Collar bone, sternum I: Front of humerus	Rotates arm towards chest, adducts arm	• Pulling the Arms (see page 95) • Rotating the Shoulder (see page 102) • Shoulder to Opposite Knee Spinal Twist (see page 105) • Side Back Bow (see page 107) • Lateral & Crossed Scissor Stretch (see pages 108 & 122) • Kneeling Cushion, Sitting Stool & Standing Cobra (see pages 118–119, 120 & 121) • Backward Arm Lever (see page 127) • Stretching the Arm in the Triangle Position (see page 128) • Elbow Pivot Lever (see page 128) • Butterfly Shoulder Stretch (see page 131) • Feet to Back Stretch (see page 132)
Rectus abdominis	Abdomen Lessons 3, 6, 7 & 8	O: Top of pubic bone I: Cartilages of 5th, 6th, 7th ribs	Flexes spine forwards	• The Half Bridge (see page 83) • Side Back Bow (see page 107) • Lateral & Crossed Scissor Stretch (see pages 108 & 122) • Kneeling Cushion, Sitting Stool & Standing Cobra (see pages 118–119, 120 & 121) • Feet to Back Stretch (see page 132)

Subscapularis

Pectoralis major

Rectus abdominis

Back

MUSCLE	REGION LESSON	ATTACHMENTS (origin and insertion)	MUSCLE ACTION	KEY THAI MANIPULATIONS ACTING ON THE MUSCLE
Erector spinae (Sacrospinalis) (see also page 24)	Back Lessons 2, 3, 5 & 8	O: Lower-neck (cervical) vertebrae, upper-back (thoracic) vertebrae I: Upper-cervical vertebrae, base of skull and ribs	(Both sides) Extends spine backwards. (One Side) Twists spine and flexes to one side	• Chest to Foot Thigh Pressing *(see page 61)* • 'Praying Mantis' *(see page 62)* • Rotating the Hips *(see page 78)* • Rocking & Rolling the Back *(see page 80)* • The Plough *(see page 80)* • Kneeing the Buttocks *(see page 82)* • Shinning the Thighs *(see page 82)* • The Half Bridge *(see page 83)* • Lifting Head to Straight Knees *(see page 85)* • Lifting Head to Crossed Knees *(see page 85)* • Lifting Spinal Twist *(see page 109)* • Pressing Head to Knees *(see page 130)* • Butterfly Manipulation *(see page 131)*

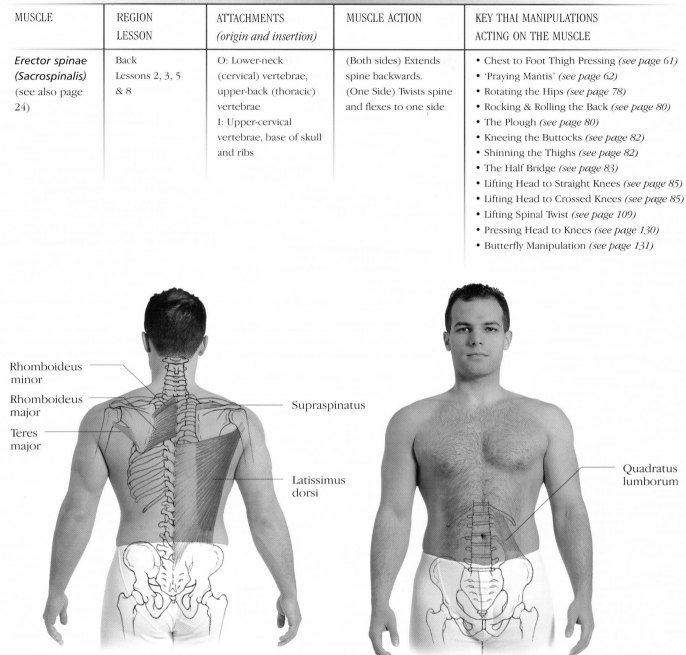

Rhomboideus minor

Rhomboideus major

Teres major

Supraspinatus

Latissimus dorsi

Quadratus lumborum

MUSCLE	REGION LESSON	ATTACHMENTS (origin and insertion)	MUSCLE ACTION	KEY THAI MANIPULATIONS ACTING ON THE MUSCLE
Latissimus dorsi	Back Lessons 3, 5, 6 & 8	O: Lower six thoracic vertebrae, lumbar vertebrae, iliac crests I: Front of humerus	Rotates arm towards chest, pulls arm backwards and inwards	• Lifting Head to Straight Knees *(see page 85)* • Lifting Head to Crossed Knees *(see page 85)* • Stretching the Arm in the Triangle Position (supine and side) *(see pages 92 & 105)* • Pulling the Arm in the Side Position *(see page 104)* • Backward Arm Lever *(see page 127)* • Elbow Pivot Lever *(see page 128)* • Seated Lateral Arm Lever *(see page 129)* • Butterfly Shoulder Stretch *(see page 131)*

MUSCLE	REGION LESSON	ATTACHMENTS (*origin and insertion*)	MUSCLE ACTION	KEY THAI MANIPULATIONS ACTING ON THE MUSCLE
Rhomboideus minor and major	Back Lessons 3, 5 & 6	O: Last cervical and first five thoracic vertebrae I: Inner margin of shoulder blade (scapula)	Pulls shoulder blades (scapula) towards spine	• Bow & Arrow Spinal Twist (*see page 78*) • Lifting Head to Straight Knees (*see page 85*) • Lifting Head to Crossed Knees (*see page 85*) • Foot to Armpit Stretch (*see page 92*) • Rotating the Shoulder (*see page 102*) • Lifting Spinal Twist (*see page 109*)
Quadratus lumborum	Back Lessons 3, 6, 7 & 8	O: Top of iliac crests I: Lumbar vertebrae and 12th rib	Sideways bending of lower back	• Bow & Arrow Spinal Twist (*see page 78*) • Stretching the Arm in the Triangle Position (*see page 105*) • Lifting Spinal Twist (*see page 109*) • Knee or Hand to Buttock/Back Backward (*see page 115*) • Seated Lateral Arm Lever (*see page 129*)

Hip and Buttock

Gluteus maximus	Buttocks Lessons 2, 3 & 6	O: Sacroiliac joint, back edge of ilium I: Below the head of femur on its posterior surface	Draws leg backwards and rotates thigh outwards	• Chest to Foot Thigh Pressing (*see page 61*) • 'Praying Mantis' (*see page 62*) • Rotating the Hip (*see page 63*) • The Plough (*see page 80*) • Kneeing the Backs of the Thighs (*see page 81*) • Shinning the Thighs (*see page 82*) • Kneeing the Buttocks (*see page 82*) • Lifting Head to Crossed Knees (*see page 85*) • Shoulder to Opposite Knee Spinal Twist (*see page 105*)

Gluteus maximus

Piriformis

Piriformis	Hips Lessons 2 & 6	O: Front surface of the sacrum I: Top of femur (great trochanter)	Draws thigh outwards, rotates thigh outwards	• 'Praying Mantis' (*see page 62*) • Rocking the Hip (*see page 68*) • Shoulder to Opposite Knee Spinal Twist (*see page 69*) • Stretching Crossed Leg Horizontally (*see page 69 and page 106*)

Legs

MUSCLE	REGION LESSON	ATTACHMENTS *(origin and insertion)*	MUSCLE ACTION	KEY THAI MANIPULATIONS ACTING ON THE MUSCLE
Psoas major	Legs Lessons 6 & 7	O: Transverse processes of all lumbar vertebrae and last thoracic vertebra I: Femur just below hip joint (lesser trochanter)	Flexes thigh up towards abdomen, flexes spine forwards	• Swinging the Legs *(see page 79)* • Knee Pivot Hip Stretch *(see page 107)* • Side Back Bow *(see page 107)* • Reverse Half Lotus Leg Lift *(see page 115)* • Knee or Hand to Buttock/Back Backward *(see page 115)* • Backward Seasaw Leg Lift *(see page 116)* • Standing Backward Leg Lift *(see page 113)* • Kneeling Cushion, Sitting Stool and Standing and Intimate Cobra *(see pages 118–119, 120 & 121)* • Lateral and Crossed Scissor Stretches *(see page 108)* • Side and Prone Positions *(see pages 99 & 123)* • Wheelbarrow *(see page 122)* • Knee to Calf Press *(see page 123)*
Iliacus	Legs Lessons 6 & 7	O: Front of iliac bones, top of sacrum I: Together with psoas major	Flexes thigh up towards abdomen	**As for psoas major**
Hamstrings: *Biceps femoris, Semitendinosus, Semimembranosus*	Legs Lessons 2, 3 & 6	O: (Biceps femoris) Ischium and posterior upper shaft of femur; (Semitendinosus and semimembranosus) ischium I: (Biceps femoris) Head of fibula; (Semitendinosus) inner surface of tibial shaft; (Semimembranosus) inner condyle of the tibia	Flexes knee, raises lower leg, rotates thigh inwards	• Chest to Foot Thigh Pressing *(see page 61)* • 'Praying Mantis' *(see page 62)* • 'Tug of War' *(see page 66)* • Pressing in the Splits Position *(see page 70)* • Half Lotus Back Rock & Roll *(see page 72)* • Vertical Half Lotus Thigh Press *(see page 72)* • Raised Foot Leg Stretch *(see page 74)* • Vertical leg Stretch *(see page 74)* • The Plough *(see page 80)* • Lifting Head to Straight Knee *(see page 85)* • Knee to Hip Flex *(see page 106)* • Stretching the Crossed Leg Horizontally *(see page 106)*
Gracilis	Legs Lessons 2 & 6	O: Lower margin of pubic bone I: Inner surface of tibial shaft	Flexes knee, rotates knee inwards, adducts thigh	• 'Tug of War' *(see page 66)* • Pressing in the Splits Position *(see page 70)* • Half Lotus Press *(see page 71)* • Half Lotus Back Rock & Roll *(see page 72)* • Corkscrew (bent leg) *(see page 73)* • Swinging the Legs *(see page 79)* • Grape Presses in all positions *(see page 100)* • Knee Pivot Hip Stretch *(see page 107)* • Knee to Buttock/Backward Leg Lift *(see page 115)*

MUSCLE	REGION LESSON	ATTACHMENTS (origin and insertion)	MUSCLE ACTION	KEY THAI MANIPULATIONS ACTING ON THE MUSCLE
Sartorius	Legs Lessons 2 & 7	O: Front of iliac bone I: Inner surface of upper tibia	Flexes thigh, rotates thigh outwards	• Pressing the Turned-in Leg (see page 67) • Lateral and Crossed Scissor Stretches (see page 108 & 122) • Standing Backward Leg Lift (see page 113) • Knee to Buttock/Backward Leg Lift (see page 115) • Reverse Half Lotus Leg Lift (see page 115) • Backward Seesaw Leg Lift (see page 116) • Wheelbarrow (see page 122)

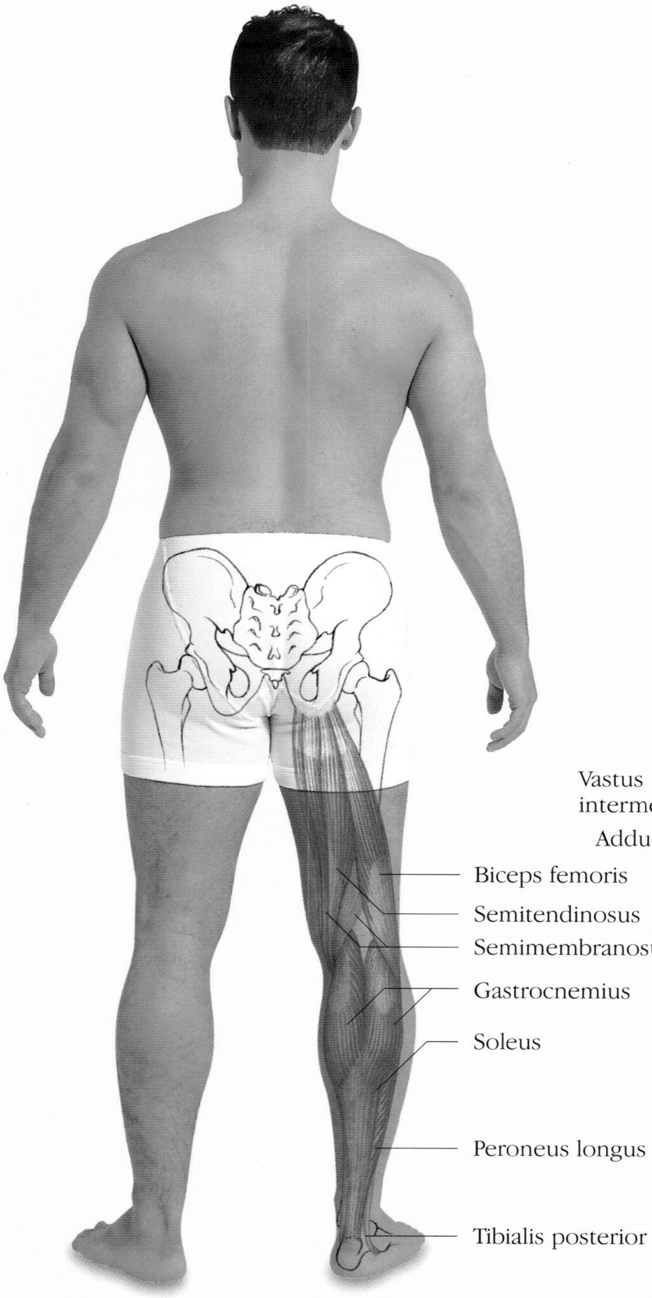

Psoas major

Iliacus

Vastus lateralis

Gracilis

Rectus femoris

Sartorius

Vastus medialis

Tibialis anterior

Vastus intermedius

Adductors

Biceps femoris

Semitendinosus

Semimembranosus

Gastrocnemius

Soleus

Peroneus longus

Tibialis posterior

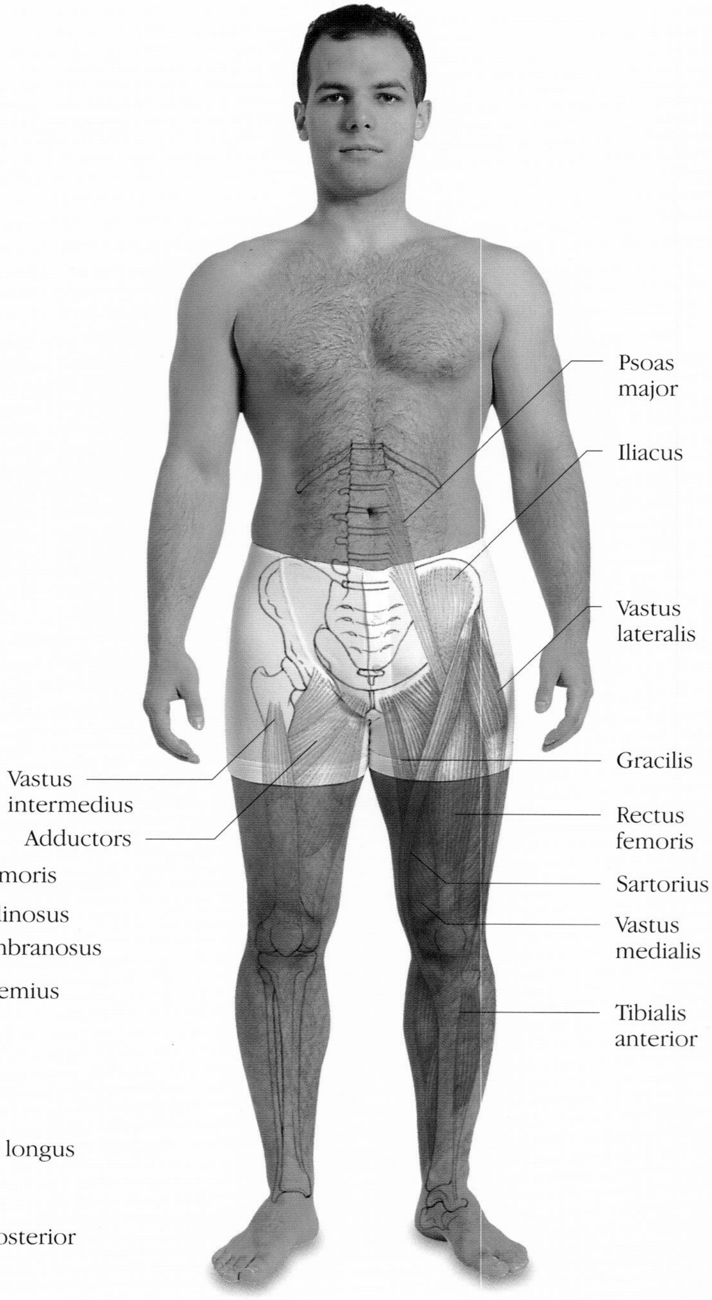

Legs continued

MUSCLE	REGION LESSON	ATTACHMENTS (origin and insertion)	MUSCLE ACTION	KEY THAI MANIPULATIONS ACTING ON THE MUSCLE
Quadriceps: Rectus femoris Vastus medialis Vastus intermedius Vastus lateralis	Legs Lessons 2, 3, 6 & 7	O: (RF) Ilium of pelvis (Vasti) Femur I: Via patellar (kneecap) ligament to tibia	Extends leg at knee, flexes thigh at hip	• 'Praying Mantis' *(see page 62)* • Pressing the Turned-in Leg *(see page 67)* • Corkscrew *(see page 73)* • The Half Bridge *(see page 83)* • Pressing the Back of the Extended Leg *(see page 99)* • Pressing the Flexed Leg *(see page 99)* • Shoulder to Opposite Knee Spinal Twist *(see page 105)* • Knee Pivot Hip Stretch *(see page 107)* • Side Back Bow *(see page 107)* • Foot Cracker *(see page 112)* • Pressing Feet to Buttock *(see page 113)* • Standing Backward Leg Lift *(see page 113)* • Reverse Half Lotus Leg Flex *(see page 114)* • Reverse Half Lotus Leg Lift *(see page 115)* • Knee to Buttock/Backward Leg Lift *(see page 115)* • Backward Seesaw Leg Lift *(see page 116)* • Wheelbarrow *(see page 122)* • Lateral and Crossed Scissor Stretches *(see pages 108 & 122)* • Knee to Calf Press *(see page 123)*

Biceps femoris

Peroneus longus

MUSCLE	REGION LESSON	ATTACHMENTS *(origin and insertion)*	MUSCLE ACTION	KEY THAI MANIPULATIONS ACTING ON THE MUSCLE
Adductors	Legs Lessons 2, 3 & 6	O: Pubic bone and ischium I: Inner margin of upper femur	Draws leg towards midline (adduction)	• Pressing the Leg in the Tree Position *(see page 56)* • Half Lotus Press *(see page 71)* • Half Lotus Back Rock & Roll *(see page 72)* • Corkscrew *(see page 73)* • Pressing in the Splits Position *(see page 70)* • Swinging the Legs *(see page 79)* • The Plough *(see page 80)* • Lifting Head to Crossed Knees *(see page 85)* • Grape Presses in all positions *(see page 100)* • Knee Pivot Hip Stretch *(see page 107)* • Lateral and Crossed Scissor Stretch *(see page 108)*
Peroneus longus	Legs Lesson 1	O: Upper, outer surface of fibula I: Base of first metatarsal	Flexes foot downwards and turns it outwards (everts)	• Pressing the Feet Sideways *(see page 45)* • Pressing the Crossed Feet *(see page 45)* • Pressing the Feet Backwards and Forwards *(see page 47)*
Tibialis anterior	Legs Lessons 1 & 7	O: Outer margin of tibia I: Base of metatarsal bones	Flexes foot upwards at ankle and turns it inwards	• Pressing Feet and Ankles *(see page 45)* • Pressing the Feet Sideways *(see page 45)* • Pressing the Feet Forwards & Backwards *(see page 45)* • Pressing the Crossed Feet *(see page 45)* • Stretching the Arched Foot *(see page 50)* • Pressing Thigh to Calf *(see page 64)* • Pressing Heel to Buttock *(see page 112)* • Pressing the Thigh & Pulling the Foot *(see page 112)* • Foot Cracker *(see page 112)* • Reverse Half Lotus Leg Flex *(see page 114)*
Tibialis posterior	Legs Lesson 1	O: Posterior of Tibia and Fibula upper shafts I: Third and fourth metatarsals	Flexes foot arch, turns foot inwards and supports the arch	• Pressing the Feet Sideways *(see page 45)* • Pressing the Feet Backwards and Forwards *(see page 47)* • Flexing the Ankle Backwards *(see page 48)*
Gastrocnemius	Legs Lessons 2, 3, 6 & 7	O: Inner surface and outer surface of lower femur I: Heel bone (calcaneus)	Extends foot downwards and flexes leg at knee	• Flexing and Stretching the Leg *(see page 65)* • Pressing in the Splits Position *(see page 70)* • Rocking & Rolling the Back *(see page 80)* • Lifting Head to Straight Knees *(see page 85)* • Vertical Leg Stretch *(see page 74)* • Stretching the Crossed Leg Horizontally *(see page 69 & 107)* • Knee to Calf Press *(see page 123)*
Soleus	Legs Lessons 1, 2, 3, 6 & 7	O: Back of upper tibia and fibula I: Heel bone (calcaneus)	Extends foot downwards	*As for gastrocnemius* • Pressing the Feet Backwards and Forwards *(see page 47)* • Flexing the Ankle Backwards *(see page 48)*

Arms & Hands

MUSCLE	REGION LESSON	ATTACHMENTS (origin and insertion)	MUSCLE ACTION	KEY THAI MANIPULATIONS ACTING ON THE MUSCLE
Biceps	Arm Lessons 3, 5 & 8	O: Scapula (two heads) I: Radius	Flexes arm at elbow	• Lifting Head to Straight Knees *(see page 85)* • Pulling the Arms *(see page 95)* • Feet to Back Stretch *(see page 132)*
Triceps	Arm Lessons 5, 6 & 8	O: Humerus (two heads), scapula I: Ulna	Extends arm at elbow	• Stretching the Arm in the Triangle Position (supine and side) *(see pages 92 & 105)* • Backward Arm Lever *(see page 127)* • Elbow Pivot Lever *(see page 128)* • Butterfly Shoulder Stretch *(see page 131)*
Wrist and hand extensors	Arm Lesson 5	O: Humerus, radius, ulna I: Wrist bones, hand bones, finger and thumb bones	Extend palms of hands backwards at wrist, and all the fingers and thumbs	• Rotating the Wrist *(see page 94)*
Wrist and hand flexors	Arm Lessons 5 & 6	O: Humerus, radius, ulna I: Wrist bones, hand bones, finger and thumb bones	Flex palms of hands upwards at wrist, and fingers and thumbs	• Stretching the Arm in the Triangle Position (supine and side) *(see pages 92 & 105)* • Knee to Hand Pressing *(see page 94)* • Rotating the Wrist *(see page 94)*

Biceps

Triceps

Flexors

Extensors

33

CHAPTER 2
THE MECHANICS OF THAI MASSAGE

To create the fundamental effect of pressure that is needed for Thai bodywork, force is applied by the masseur. 'Soft tissue massage' and 'manipulation' describe the two aspects of Thai bodywork. In soft tissue massage, pressure is used directly for the desired effect. For the manipulative techniques, pressure is used to achieve stretching and twisting. Traditional Thai bodywork massage is remarkable for the number of different positions in which the receiver's body is presented to the masseur, who also has to adopt a corresponding variety of body positions.

Many of the manipulations in Thai bodywork involve substantial leverage. This often works to the advantage of the practitoner by enabling a small effort to achieve a large effect. This will also benefit the receiver provided that care is taken to avoid overstretching which could occur if manipulations were performed hastily.

Soft Tissue Pressure Techniques

Pressing is the basis of all soft tissue massage techniques. Skilful application of pressure can affect different levels within the tissues and enhances the flow of energy. The application of a force through a larger body surface, such as the palm or the sole of the foot, creates a pressure which is spread out and does not penetrate too deeply. If the same force is applied with the thumb or the tip of the elbow to cover a smaller area, a much more focused and penetrating pressure results. For all pressure techniques, always start with light pressing and increase gradually. Some people find very deep pressure extremely painful.

• SINGLE THUMB PRESSING

In the single thumb pressing method, pressure is always applied using the pad of the thumb. The tip of the thumb is never used. Thai bodywork is unique in frequently combining thumb pressing while stretching a body part at the same time. Pressing affects the underlying tissues in a way that makes them more amenable to the flow of energy and the drainage of lymph.

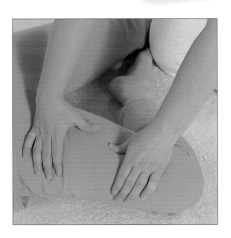

• THUMB WALKING

This method is used to stimulate the energy channels *(see page 14)*. Movement can be in either direction along the lines. The thumbs are placed with their tips almost touching and pressed alternately as they progress along the energy lines. If movement is towards the left, the left thumb is lifted and moved two to three centimetres to the left and pressure is applied. The right thumb is then moved up to join the left and pressed in turn.

This sequence is repeated over and over again so that alternate thumb pressure is applied along the whole length of the energy lines. The 'walking' can, of course, be done from left to right.

• PALM PRESSING

The palmar surface of the hand is extensively used for applying strong pressure over larger areas of the body than would be possible with the thumbs. Pressure can be applied and sustained without movement either for a few seconds or up to several minutes. Palmar pressing can be used to create a rocking action and this is achieved with short duration presses. The upper body weight over the arms is used to generate strong and sustained pressure. To achieve the effect required without fatigue, the arms are usually kept straight. There are three different ways of pressing with the palmar surface – Single Palm Pressing, Double Palm Pressing and Butterfly Palm Pressing as follows:

CAUTION!

For all pressure techniques, start with light pressing and gradually increase.

Single Palm Pressing: The emphasis is often on the heel of the hand and this technique is used for applying firm pressure to the major soft tissue masses of the body, such as the back, buttocks and thighs.

Double Palm Pressing: Here, concentrating the pressure is achieved by placing one hand directly on top of the other.

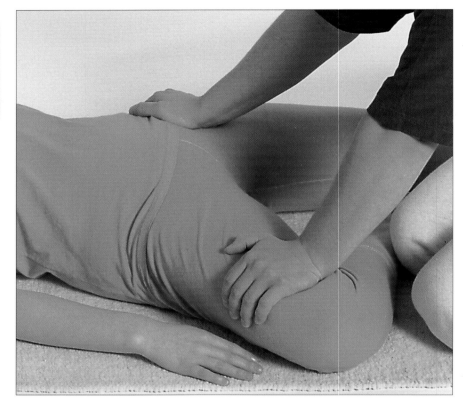

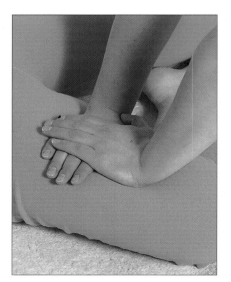

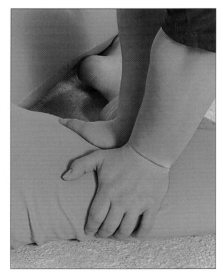

Butterfly Palm Pressing: This method involves simultaneous pressure using both hands with the heels of the palms touching. It spreads the force over an even wider area of the body.

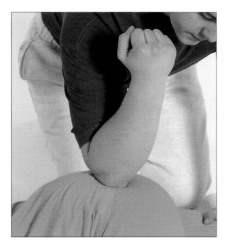

• ELBOW PRESSING

Elbow pressing with the tip of the elbow enables the masseur to apply deeper pressure than is possible with the hand. It is used on the thighs, buttocks and upper shoulders, where the muscles are thick. If the elbow tip causes too much pain, the upper forearm can be used instead to spread the force and to reduce pressure.

• KNEE PRESSING

Knee pressing frees the hands for controlling stretches while, at the same time, exerting deep pressure. It is used mainly on the backs of the legs and buttocks.

CAUTION!

For all pressure techniques, start with light pressing and gradually increase.

• FOOT PRESSING

The foot is ideally shaped to apply pressure over large areas of the body. On strongly curved parts, such as thighs, the arch is used but for thickly muscled buttocks and similar muscular areas, the heel or the front of the sole can create strong, penetrating pressure.

Some manipulations require that parts of the body are pulled against the foot to give a powerful stretch against foot pressure.

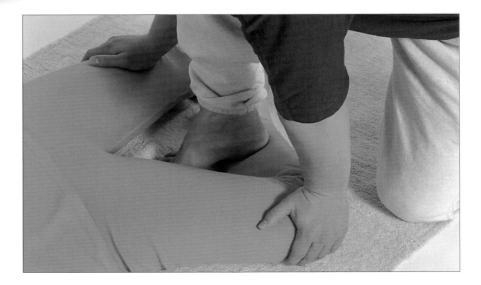

• BUTTOCK PRESSING

Controlled sitting, where more or less of the weight is taken on the practitioner's feet or knees, is sometimes applied. This is particularly useful as a means of anchoring one part of the body during a manipulation.

CAUTION!

For all pressure techniques, start with light pressing and gradually increase.

• STANDING PRESSURE

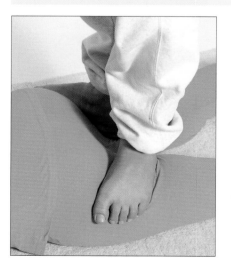

Foot pressure from a standing position can be extremely penetrating and should be applied with great care. It is used on the back, buttocks, legs and feet.

THE BENEFITS OF PRESSING

Pressure sense organs in the skin produce pleasurable sensations when subjected to large scale and sustained pressing. Too much pressure, however, creates discomfort or pain. Concentrated pressure on the energy channels boosts energy flow and deep pressure on the tissues encourages the release of adhesions in the connective tissue (myofascia) that surrounds the muscles. Blood flow in superficial capillaries and lymphatic drainage is also aided by all kinds of pressing.

Manipulation Techniques

Manipulation is the controlled movement of one or more parts of the body relative to others to achieve specific effects such as stretching and twisting.

It always involves leverage. The masseur must have a high sensitivity to its effectiveness which can result in very powerful stretches and twists with relatively little effort. A lack of this sensitivity could result in injury. In order to avoid serious back strain caused by lifting and moving in the wrong way, the giver should also be constantly aware of his/her own posture and position relative to the receiver.

• STRETCHING

The Vertical Leg Stretch is a manipulation which involves powerful leverage. A careless or insensitive masseur could easily overstretch the hamstring, gluteal and even the lower back muscles of the receiver. Always watch your partner's expression, which will quickly react to even a hint of overstretching.

THE BENEFITS OF MANIPULATIONS

Thai manipulations work on the theory that to be effective, the manipulation must always take the movement just a little further than the recipient would be capable of doing themselves unaided. A good Thai practitioner always knows exactly how far a movement can be taken without causing pain or injury to the recipient. Regular Thai bodywork progressively develops a degree of flexibility and mobility in the body which many recipients find miraculous.

With Thai manipulations there is a complex interaction between giver and receiver. This allows certain parts of the body to be reached that other forms of massage leave untreated.

Preparation for Manipulation

All the different parts of the body are manipulated during Thai bodywork and manipulation is achieved through pulling, pushing, lifting, shaking and rotating. The end result of these manipulations is stretching and twisting.

So very impressive are the Thai manipulations that the therapist can be tempted to emphasize them at the expense of pressing techniques. This is a serious mistake. Pressure on the soft tissues prepares the receiver physiologically so that the greatest benefit can be derived from the manipulations that follow them. It is the pressure techniques that are most effective in the treatment of pain and in stimulating the flow of energy in the Sen channels.

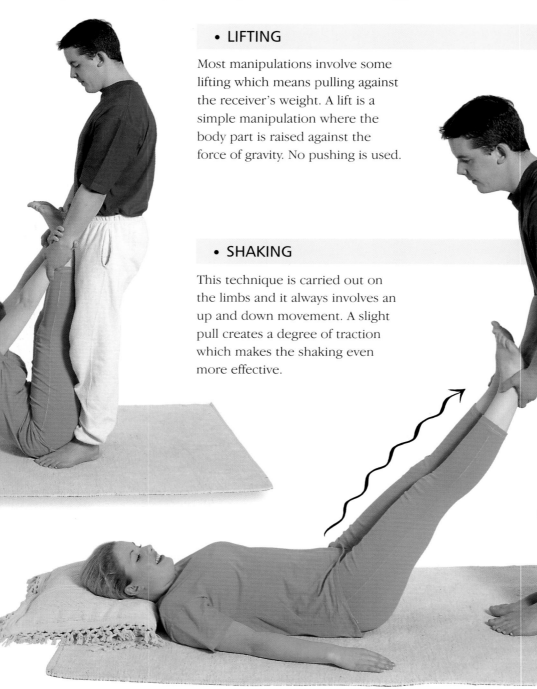

• LIFTING

Most manipulations involve some lifting which means pulling against the receiver's weight. A lift is a simple manipulation where the body part is raised against the force of gravity. No pushing is used.

• SHAKING

This technique is carried out on the limbs and it always involves an up and down movement. A slight pull creates a degree of traction which makes the shaking even more effective.

• ROTATION

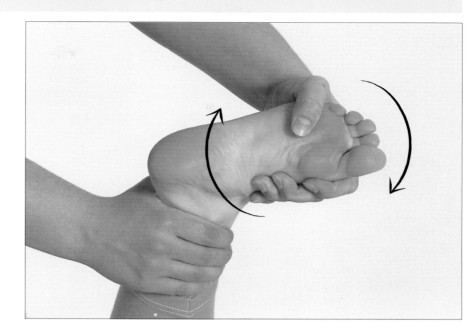

This is a 360° movement about joints such as the wrists, ankles, shoulders, hips and neck. It is the result of alternate pushing and pulling techniques. Even joints affected by osteoarthritis can have normal mobility restored through regular rotation.

• PULLING AND PUSHING

Whenever a body part is pulled, it must be anchored at its other end. Sometimes the subject's body weight achieves this. However, the strongest pulling often requires an opposing push. Thai therapists frequently use their feet for this. The most powerful sustained pulls are achieved when the practitioner's body weight is used to generate the effort. Leaning away from the subject creates this effect.

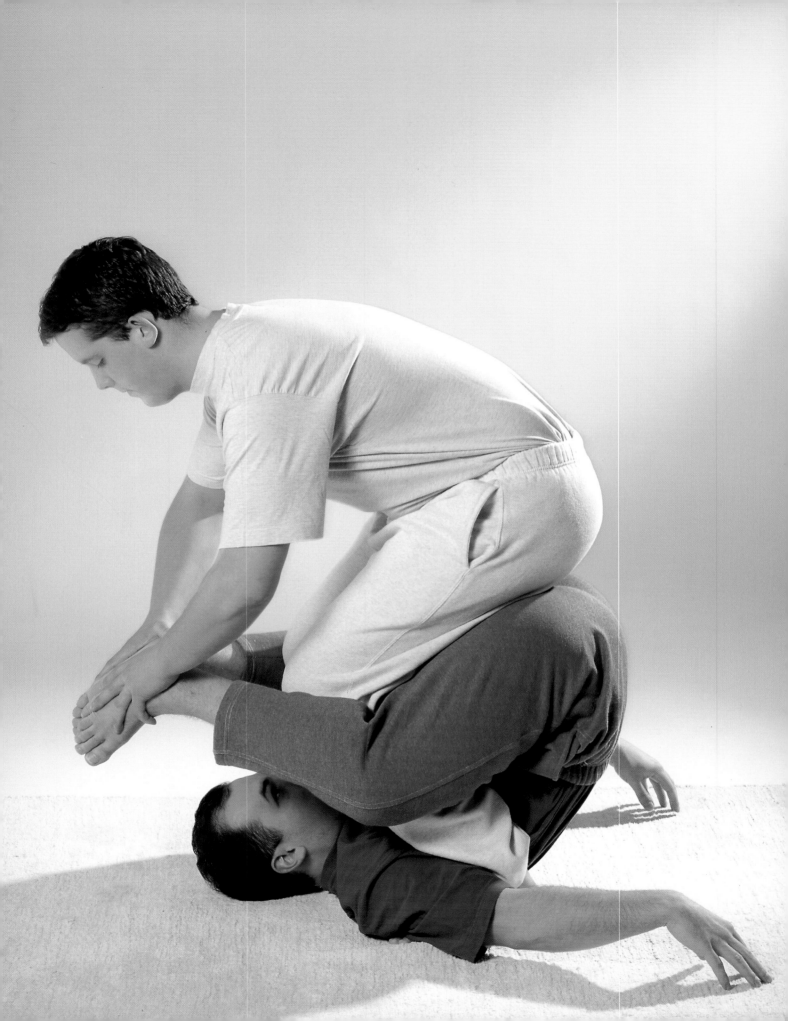

PART TWO

THAI BODYWORK PROGRAMME

The sequence shown presents a unique, whole body programme devised by Maria Mercati and based on a synthesis of techniques from northern and southern Thailand. In Thailand there are many subtle variations in both the techniques and the massage sequence.

Each step is demonstrated by a photograph; some photos have arrows superimposed to show you exactly where to apply pressure, and the healing benefits and key muscles used in each massage are listed alongside. Caution boxes indicate where you should take care with a particular technique, but it should be emphasized here again that Thai massage is not recommended during pregnancy.

The Thai Massage Routine

LESSON	POSITION OF SUBJECT	PART OF BODY MASSAGED
One	Supine (Lying on the back)	a) Both feet simultaneously b) Each foot individually
Two	Supine	a) Both feet and legs simultaneously b) Left leg only c) Right leg only
Three	Supine	Both legs simultaneously and back
Four	Supine	a) Abdomen b) Chest
Five	Supine	a) Arms and hands individually b) Face, neck, shoulders and head
Six	Lying on the left or right side	Repetition of all parts of the body that can be reached in the side position. (Note: The left side is a mirror image of the right side.)
Seven	Prone (lying face downwards)	a) Legs b) Back c) Arms
Eight	Sitting	a) Shoulders and neck b) Face c) Head

Lesson One

THE FEET

T*he massage starts here and, since this is the first physical contact between the giver and receiver, the scene should be set very carefully (see page 17). To receive massage, your partner should be lying very comfortably in the supine position (lying on the back) with arms in a relaxed position down the sides of the body, and with legs apart leaving a gap of one body-width between the feet.*

The aim of Lesson One is to stimulate the smooth energy flow through the Sen (energy lines) of the feet and legs. Refer to Part One Chapter Two (see pages 34–41) for the basic techniques of pressing and manipulation.

Sen channels on the feet

There are five Sen channels on the soles of the feet. They all start at a point on the front margin of the heel pad on the mid line. The Sen channels radiate from this point to the toes.

Thumb press from the centre heel point towards each toe, working both feet together. Press the Sen channels as many times as the strength of your thumb permits. Feet bear the weight of the whole body as well as moving to walk and run, so they require both flexibility and strength. Working through the techniques in this lesson will help your partner maintain foot flexibility and avoid injury.

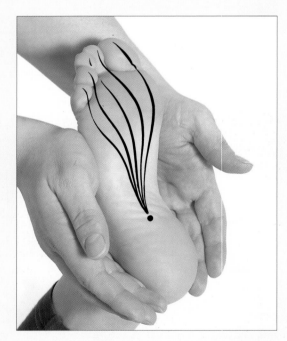

ABOVE: *These are the five Sen on the soles of the foot. Thorough pressing of these Sen is regarded as a vital prelude to overall energy balance.*

Massaging both feet

1 PRESSING FEET & ANKLES

Kneeling between your partner's legs, grasp both feet. Keep your arms straight so that your body weight can be transferred through them. Rock forward and outwards or from side to side, increasing pressure through the palms. Move your palms down the inner margins of her feet towards her toes using pressure at each position.

HEALING BENEFITS

- *Warms and loosens the feet, and has a relaxing effect on the recipient.*
- *Twists the thighs outwards and exercises the hip.*

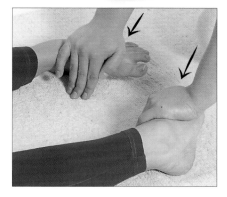

2 PRESSING THE FEET SIDEWAYS

Press your partner's feet outwards (evert) as far as they will stretch and hold them in place for a few seconds. Release her feet, place your hands across the top part of the feet and press them inwards (invert) as shown, left. Repeat the sequence once or twice.

HEALING BENEFITS

- *Improves ankle flexibility.*

3 PRESSING THE CROSSED FEET

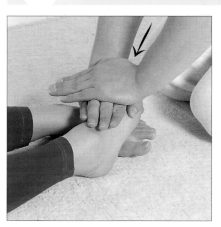

Bring your partner's feet together to cross one foot over the other. Apply gentle sustained downward pressure on them, then reverse positions and press again.

HEALING BENEFITS

- *Loosens the ankles, arches and toes, so increasing the flexibility of the tarso-metatarsal joints.*

MUSCLES STRETCHED & PRESSED

- 1. PRESSING FEET & ANKLES
  Stretched: *Tibialis anterior (outwards)*

- 2. PRESSING THE FEET SIDEWAYS
  Stretched: *Tibialis anterior (outwards), tibialis posterior (inwards), peroneus longus (inwards)*

- 3. PRESSING THE CROSSED FEET
  Stretched: *Peroneus longus, tibialis posterior*

45

4   SQUEEZING THE FEET

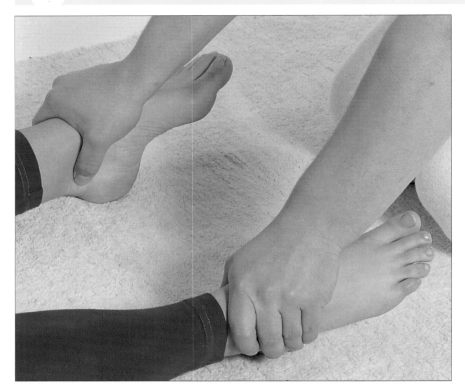

Grasp the tops of your partner's feet and squeeze firmly and progressively down towards the toes. Repeat several times.

HEALING BENEFITS

• *Improves flexibility of the feet.*

5   FLICKING THE TOES

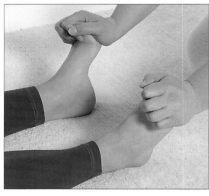

Place the heel of your hand under your partner's toes and close your fingers above all the toes. Slide your hands off the toes, flicking them upwards as you do so. Then repeat Technique 1.

HEALING BENEFITS

• *Produces a pleasant, relaxing sensation for the recipient.*

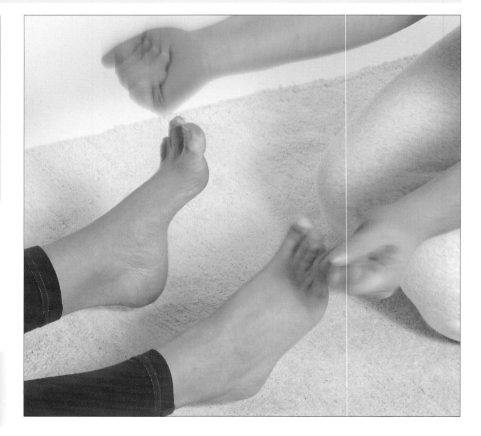

6 PRESSING THE FEET BACKWARDS & FORWARDS

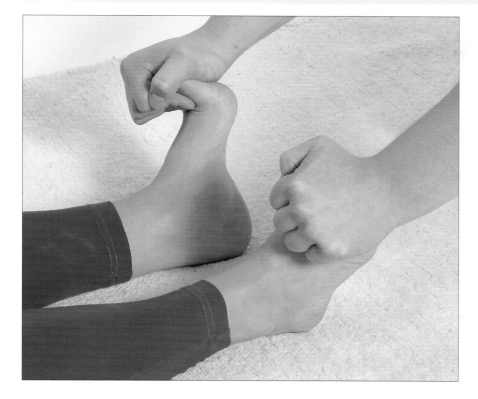

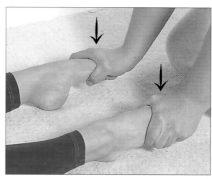

Place the heels of your palms under your partner's toes and firmly push towards her head. Then with your palms on top of the toes, press downwards.

HEALING BENEFITS

• *Improves flexibility of the ankles and the feet.*

7 PRESSING POINTS ON ANKLES & FEET

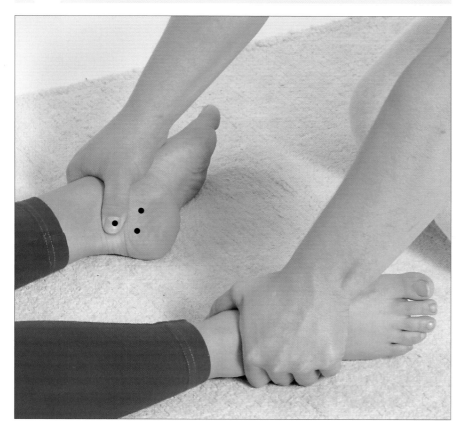

MUSCLES STRETCHED & PRESSED

• 6. PRESSING THE FEET BACKWARDS & FORWARDS
Stretched: *Peroneus longus (upward), tibialis posterior (upward), soleus (upward), tibialis anterior (downward)*

Thumb press deeply into the three ankle points, marked here with dots, on both your partner's feet *(see left)*. Then thumb press around the margins of the undersides of her heels. Now thumb press along the energy lines between her heel and toes *(see page 38)*.

HEALING BENEFITS

• *Balances the energies within the reproductive system and organs of the lower back.*

Massaging each foot individually

1   FLEXING THE ANKLE BACKWARDS

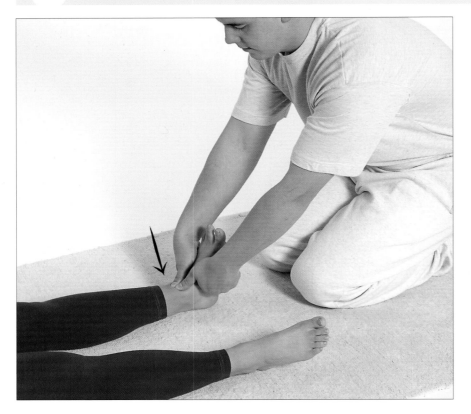

Grasp your partner's foot with both hands, pressing your thumbs down into the centre of her front ankle crease. Then lean forward to press her foot backwards against this pressure.

HEALING BENEFITS

• *Increases flexibility of the ankle.*
• *Beneficial for those who suffer from headaches.*

2   PRESSING THE TENDONS OF THE UPPER FOOT

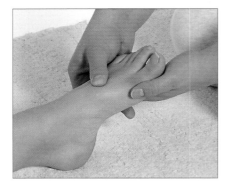

With circular movements, thumb press into the spaces between your partner's tendons. Begin at the hollow at the centre of the top of each ankle and work your way towards her toes. Follow each tendon in turn.

HEALING BENEFITS

• *Has an invigorating effect upon the recipient.*
• *Increases blood flow around the tendons (tissue which is normally very inert) which helps to maintain healthy feet.*

3   PULLING & CRACKING EACH TOE

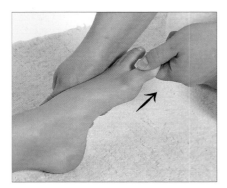

Hold each of your partner's toes, lean back and pull vigorously in turn. During this technique a cracking sound may be heard.

HEALING BENEFITS

• *Loosens toe joints and increases blood circulation.*

4   TWISTING THE FEET

Support your partner's foot with one hand and bend the free edge of her foot up and down with a twisting, flicking action. Do this two to three times whilst working towards her toes. Repeat the sequence on the opposite side of her foot.

HEALING BENEFITS

• *Stimulates the foot and increases lateral flexibility.*
• *The intrinsic muscles of the foot are well stretched during the twisting movements.*

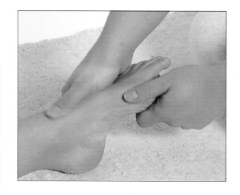

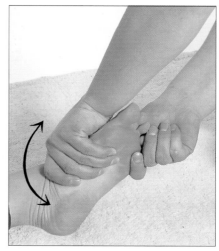

5   MASSAGING THE TOES

Touch Method One: Fast Toe Pulling Start by rapidly pulling all your partner's toes. Use all your fingers simultaneously and work with a rapid snapping action as the toes are released.

Touch Method Two: Rotating & Squeezing Rotate each of your partner's toes both ways. Follow this with a firm squeezing action towards the tip of the toes and release with a sliding movement.

MUSCLES STRETCHED & PRESSED

• 1. FLEXING THE ANKLE BACKWARDS
Stretched: *Peroneus longus (upward), tibialis posterior (upward), soleus.*

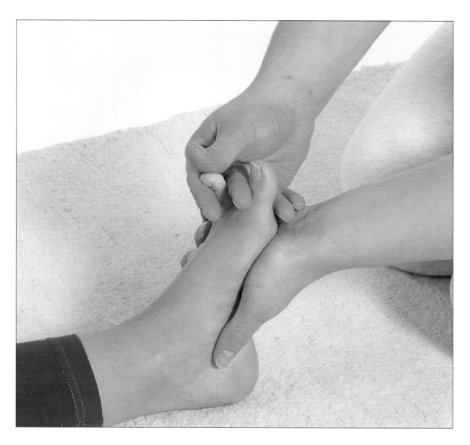

Touch Method Three: Toe Tip Massage Here, the toe is held between two fingers and the extreme tip is massaged vigorously with a circular motion.

HEALING BENEFITS

• *Brings the recipient's awareness into the tips of the toes which is both stimulating and relaxing.*
• *Starting points of the Sen channels are massaged to affect overall energy balance very positively.*

6   STRETCHING THE ARCHED FOOT

Grasp your partner's foot with your thumbs over the front of her ankle. Lean back as you press down with the base of your thumbs to stretch her foot into an arched position. Repeat this stretch twice: first, with your hands around her instep and then again nearer her toes which are arched downwards.

HEALING BENEFITS

• *Improves the lateral flexibility of the foot and strengthens the instep.*

7   ROTATING THE FOOT

While supporting your partner's leg above the ankle, firmly grasp her foot from below and rotate it several times in both directions.

HEALING BENEFITS

• *Improves flexibility of the ankles.*

8   ROTATING THE HEEL

Grasp your partner's heel as shown and then rotate it with a simultaneous squeezing action.

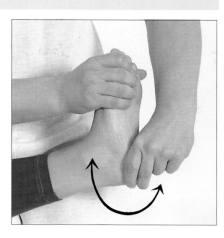

MUSCLES STRETCHED & PRESSED

- 6. STRETCHING THE ARCHED FOOT
  Stretched: *Foot flexors, tibialis anterior*

- 7. ROTATING THE FOOT
  Stretched: *Soleus, foot extensors and flexors*

9   PRESSING THE FOOT SEN

Grasp your partner's foot in both hands so that your fingertips are lined up along the energy channels *(see page 38)* on the sole. Using the fingers of both your hands simultaneously, dig your fingertips right into the sole and press deeply with a squeezing action into the central and then the two lateral Sen channels in turn. Then thumb press along all five Sen channels.

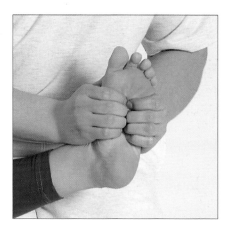

HEALING BENEFITS

- *Promotes improved foot flexibility and stimulates Sen energy flow.*

10   PUMMELLING THE HEEL

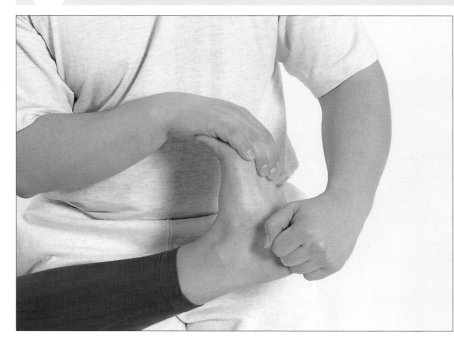

Stretching your partner's toes towards her head, pummel the underside of her heel using your clenched fist.

Now repeat Techniques 1–10 as described above on her other foot.

HEALING BENEFITS

- *Stimulates energy flow in the feet, creating a feeling of groundedness.*

Lesson Two

THE FEET & LEGS

The first part of Lesson Two is a prelude to the more intensive leg manipulations which follow. Refer to Part One Chapter Two (see pages 34–41) for the basic techniques of pressing and manipulation. The receiver lies in the supine position (lying on the back) and each leg is held straight and thoroughly pressed using the palms and thumbs. Ensure that all the Sen channels are equally stimulated along the entire length of the leg.

In the second part of Lesson Two, the leg is placed in every position possible to give complete access to the Sen (see below right). The techniques are applied first to one leg and then repeated on the other.

Sen channels on the legs

Energy balance in the leg Sen is essential for energy balance in the spine. Throughout the bodywork, Thais place much emphasis on the legs as energy flow through them strongly affects the health of the upper body. There is no general agreement as to the exact course of the Sen channels or even the precise number but many experts consider there to be three lines on the inside and three on the outside of each leg. This corresponds to the Chinese energy meridians, the exact courses of which have been confirmed by Russian scientists.

Inside Leg Sen Channels

The Sen channels on the inside of the leg are located as follows:

• ① – Chinese Spleen meridian. This begins under the inner ankle bone and runs just along the inner edge of the shin bone to just beneath the knee. It then runs up the thigh to the top of the groin.

• ② – Chinese Liver meridian. This starts in front of the inner ankle bone and runs up the middle of the inner side of the calf muscle to just below the knee level. It restarts above the knee and runs roughly parallel with channel ① to the groin.

• ③ – Chinese Kidney meridian. This begins between the Achilles tendon and the inner ankle bone and runs along the calf to a point just on the back knee crease. It continues above the knee to deep inside the groin.

Outside Leg Sen channels

Sen channels on the outside of the leg are located as follows:

• ① – Chinese Stomach meridian. This starts on the front of the ankle and runs parallel to the outer edge of the shin bone (tibia) to a point just below the knee. It restarts on the thigh just above and in line with the outer edge of the patella, and runs directly towards the hip joint.

• ② – Chinese Gallbladder meridian. This begins on the lower front edge of the ankle bone and runs towards the side of the knee diverging slightly from channel ① as it goes. It restarts on the side of the thigh, about one thumb-width behind channel ① and runs roughly parallel to it towards the hip joint.

• ③ – Chinese Bladder meridian. This starts between the Achilles tendon and the outer ankle bone. It runs up the midline of the back of the calf and continues up the back midline of the thigh.

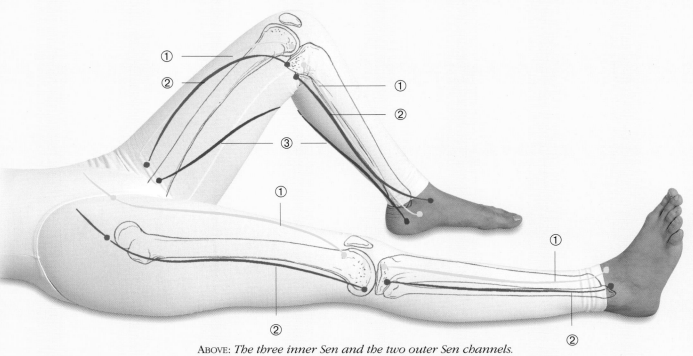

ABOVE: *The three inner Sen and the two outer Sen channels. The third outer Sen channel is under the straight leg and cannot be seen in this position.*

Pressing the legs

1 PRESSING THE INNER FEET & LEGS

Simultaneously palm press your partner's feet and ankles, rocking them outwards or from side to side. Then proceed up the inner margin of her legs to the groin, and back again. Do not press her knee directly but lightly rub it. Repeat several times.

Remember to maintain an even rhythm as sharp discontinuities in the technique will spoil the relaxing flow for the recipient.

HEALING BENEFITS

- *Loosens hip joints and unblocks the Sen channels in both legs.*
- *The gentle rocking motion has a pleasantly calming effect on your partner.*

2 PRESSING THE INNER RIGHT LEG

Touch Method One: Palm Pressing Kneel between your partner's legs facing the inside of her right leg. Starting above and below her right knee, palm press with both hands simultaneously up the thigh and down the calf, and then return.

You could also start just above the ankle using both hands side by side and gradually palm press up the leg and down again. Repeat, palm-pressing each Sen channel.

HEALING BENEFITS

- *Assists myofascial release and stimulates energy flow in the Sen.*

3 PRESSING THE OUTER RIGHT LEG

Now change position to outside the right leg and repeat the palming and thumbing sequences on the outer energy lines of your partner's right leg. Repeat on the left leg.

HEALING BENEFITS

• *Assists the flow of energy in the legs and can also relieve sciatic pain.*

MUSCLES STRETCHED & PRESSED

• 1. PRESSING THE INNER FEET & LEGS
   Stretched: *Soleus, gastrocnemius, adductors*

• 2. PRESSING THE INNER RIGHT LEG
   Stretched: *Soleus, gastrocnemius, adductors*

• 3. PRESSING THE OUTER RIGHT LEG
   Stretched: *Peroneus longus, gastrocnemius, biceps femoris, vastus lateralis*

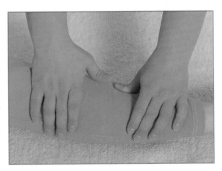

Touch Method Two: Thumb Pressing
Using the thumb walking technique, thumb up Sen channel ① to your partner's knee, down line ② to her ankle, up line ③ to her knee and down line two again. Repeat this sequence several times.

When you have finished thumbing the lower leg, move up and repeat the sequence on the upper Sen channels spanning the knee to the groin. Finish by palming her leg once more.

Massaging the right leg only

1 PRESSING THE LEG IN THE TREE POSITION

Touch Method One Place your partner's right leg in the tree position, keeping the foot tucked against her straight leg. Support her left hip with your right hand while you palm up and down the inner Sen channels of the bent leg with a slight rocking action. Do not hurry your movements – the presses should be sustained.

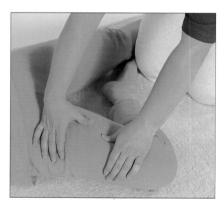

Touch Method Two: Thumb Pressing Proceed from palming to thumbing, which is carried out in exactly the same way as described earlier *(see page 35)*.

HEALING BENEFITS

• *Aids flexibility and relaxation of the knee and hip.*
• *Promotes energy flow in channels that affect the urino-genital organs.*

2 BUTTERFLY PRESSING THE LEG IN THE TREE POSITION

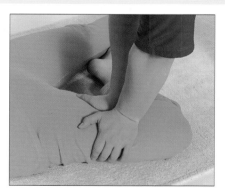

Slightly alter your position facing directly towards your partner's flexed knee. Using both hands simultaneously, butterfly press the entire length of the flexed leg.

HEALING BENEFITS

• *Even the stiffest hips and knees can be coaxed into a state of relaxation and release.*
• *Especially helpful for those who experience spasms and stiffness in the adductor muscles of the thigh.*

3 FOOT PRESSING THE LEG IN THE TREE POSITION

Touch Method One Assume a kneeling stance, balancing yourself by lightly leaning on your partner's thigh and knee. Use your right foot to massage her bent leg. Press carefully and deeply all along her thigh with your toes and the ball of your foot. Rock forward slowly to attain the necessary pressure.

HEALING BENEFITS

• *Tight and spasming thigh adductor muscles respond well to the foot pressing methods.*

HEALING BENEFITS

• *Helps tight or spasming calf muscles to relax, stimulating blood and lymph flow.*
• *Treats calf muscle sports injuries.*

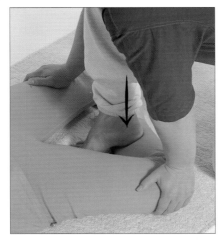

Touch Method Two With a slight change in your position, heel press along your partner's calf muscles using your body weight to achieve controlled pressure.

MUSCLES STRETCHED & PRESSED

• 1. PRESSING THE LEG IN THE TREE POSITION

• 2. BUTTERFLY PRESSING THE LEG IN THE TREE POSITION

• 3. FOOT PRESSING THE LEG IN THE TREE POSITION
Stretched: *Adductors, sartorius*
Pressed: *Adductors, soleus, gracilis, semimembranosus, semitendinosus, gastrocnemius*

- *These powerful techniques relax the inner hamstrings, enhance knee mobility and boost Sen energies.*
- *Some types of sciatica are eased.*
- *Useful for treating hamstrings injured through sport.*

4 'SINGLE GRAPE PRESS'

Place the sole of your left foot against your partner's right thigh just behind and above the knee Hold both of her feet and lean back while you press up the thigh towards the groin and back again as if you were treading grapes.

5 'SINGLE GRAPE PRESS & TWISTED VINE'

Now tuck your left foot snugly behind your partner's knee and cross her leg across your shin, tucking her toes behind your knee to give the impression of a twisted vine. Hold her heel to keep the foot in this position while you bring your right foot across and place it under her right thigh. Now press progressively with your right foot towards her groin and back again keeping a steady slow rhythm and firm pressure. Repeat several times.

6 'DOUBLE GRAPE PRESS'

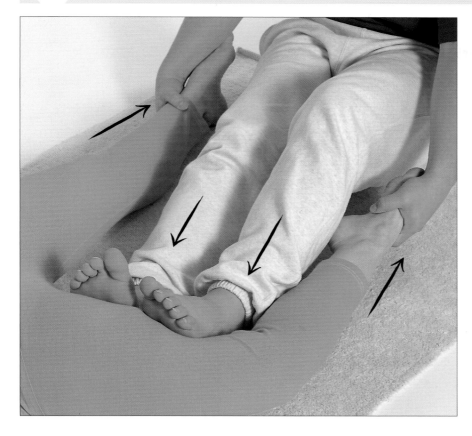

Release your partner's right foot from the locked position but continue to hold her ankles. Now press up and down her thigh using your feet alternately. Repeat several times.

MUSCLES STRETCHED & PRESSED

- 4. 'SINGLE GRAPE PRESS'
  Stretched: *Adductors, sartorius, gracilis*
  Pressed: *Adductors, hamstrings*

- 5. 'SINGLE GRAPE PRESS & TWISTED VINE'
  Stretched: *Adductors, sartorius, gracilis*
  Pressed: *Adductors, hamstrings*

- 6. 'DOUBLE GRAPE PRESS'
  Stretched: *Adductors, sartorius, gracilis*
  Pressed: *Adductors, hamstrings*

- 7. 'GRAPE PRESS & SQUEEZE'
  Stretched: *Thigh adductors, sartorius, gracilis*
  Pressed: *Adductors, hamstrings*

7 'GRAPE PRESS & SQUEEZE'

Now place your right foot on your partner's inner thigh and slide your left foot under the leg. Squeeze and press both the inner and outer thighs together. Start at the knee, pressing and squeezing up the thigh and then back to the knee. Lean your body back with each press and squeeze.

8 'Z-STOP'

Keep your feet tucked in snugly behind your partner's knee and cross her lower leg across both your shins. Her leg will become bent at a sharply acute angle that resembles a 'Z' shape *(below)*. Slide forward a little to grasp the front surface of her thigh and pull it towards you. Pull alternately with both hands along the length of her thigh *(below right)*.

HEALING BENEFITS

- *Promotes limb relaxation, increased hip and knee flexibility.*
- *Stimulates the energy channels.*

9 PULLING THE CALF

Touch Method One Lift your partner's flexed leg and lock her foot between your knees. Place your hands behind her calf muscle and pull it towards you, rocking gently backwards. Repeat at different positions along the calf moving towards the ankle. Repeat. *Touch Method Two* Place your left hand behind your partner's upper calf muscle. Squeeze and simultaneously drag the muscle to your left. Change hands and repeat in the opposite direction.

HEALING BENEFITS

- *Stimulates energy flow in the central Sen channel to ease fibrotic and adhesive connective tissue.*
- *Good for football and rugby players.*

10 PRESSING THE UPPER THIGH

Touch Method One Interlock the fingers of both your hands and place them across the top of your partner's thigh just above the top of her knee *(below)*. Squeeze firmly with the heels of your hands to cover the full length of the upper leg to the groin. Repeat several times.

Touch Method Two Pummel inner and outer thighs and calves at the same time. Repeat several times.

HEALING BENEFITS

- *Powerful myofascial release occurs and the energy flow in the major channels is unblocked.*
- *Benefits sciatica sufferers.*

MUSCLES STRETCHED & PRESSED

- 8. 'Z-STOP'
  Stretched: *Quadriceps, adductors*
  Pressed: *Hamstrings, adductors, quadriceps*

- 9. PULLING THE CALF
  Pressed: *Gastrocnemius, soleus*

- 10. PRESSING THE UPPER THIGH
  Pressed: *Quadriceps, sartorius, gracilis, semimembranosus*

- 11. CHEST TO FOOT THIGH PRESSING
  Stretched: *Gluteus maximus, quadriceps, erector spinae*
  Pressed: *Hamstrings*

11 CHEST TO FOOT THIGH PRESSING

Lift your partner's right leg and place her foot on your chest. Support her knee with your right hand and, with your left hand, press firmly into the thigh muscles. Gently rock her in a forwards-and-backwards motion as you press up and down the thigh muscle.

HEALING BENEFITS

- *Gives myofascial release to the hamstring group of muscles.*
- *Eases hip pain and sciatica.*

Touch Method One Slide your partner's foot into the area of your left groin. Stabilize her right knee with your left hand and with your right hand, palmar press your way along the inner margin of her thigh. Pressure applied in this way will force the leg outward into an everted position, but you should only attempt to press it onto the floor if your partner is very flexible.

Touch Method Two Swing your partner's knee *(right)* across her left hip. Use your right hand to keep it in position and palmar press the outer margin of her thigh with your left hand.
Note: In both of these positions, pressure should be applied rhythmically and progressively through smooth to-and-fro rocking movements (like the characteristic motion of a praying mantis insect).

13 ROTATING THE HIP

Hold your partner's ankle with your right hand and support the top of her knee with your left. Lean forward and rotate her thigh using small, circular movements, increasing to larger circles but without causing pain.

HEALING BENEFITS

• *Improves flexibility of hip points, arthritic hips, pain in the groin area associated with sciatica and lower back pain.*

MUSCLES STRETCHED & PRESSED

• 12. 'PRAYING MANTIS'
Stretched: *Adductors, gluteals, erector spinae, quadriceps piriformis*
Pressed: *Semimembranosus, semitendinosus, biceps femoris, vastus lateralis*

• 13. ROTATING THE HIP
Stretched: *Gluteus maximus, piriformis, sacrospinalis, quadriceps*

• 14. KNEEING THE THIGH
Pressed: *Hamstrings*

14 KNEEING THE THIGH

Lift your partner's right leg and place your left knee against the back of her thigh. Hold her heel and knee and, with a gentle action, pull her thigh against your knee. Relax the pulling force, lower your knee slightly and pull again. Repeat several times to knee-press progressively the entire length of the back thigh.

HEALING BENEFITS

• *Good for the treatment of tense and spasming hamstrings caused by sports injury, repetitive strain, back pain and sciatica.*

63

15 PRESSING THIGH TO CALF

With your left knee directed towards your partner's right leg, place the calf of her right leg across your thigh. Press down on her knee and foot. Adjust the position of her leg to press the whole of her calf progressively.

HEALING BENEFITS

• *Assists myofascial release in the calf muscles and eases the tension and spasming that can be caused by sports injury.*

16 'ARM CRACKER'

Tuck your left wrist and forearm tightly in behind your partner's knee. Now press her foot downwards to give a very strong stretch across the entrapped arm. Repeat two to three times.

HEALING BENEFITS

• *Treats knee pain, spasming hamstring and calf muscles.*

17 FLEXING & STRETCHING THE LEG

Grasp your partner's right heel underneath and support the side of her knee. Flex her leg at the knee by pushing the knee and then sharply extend it to maximum effect by pulling the heel, assisted by a quick pull on the knee. Repeat this exercise several times.

MUSCLES STRETCHED & PRESSED

- 15. PRESSING THIGH TO CALF
  Stretched: *Anterior tibialis*
  Pressed: *Gastrocnemius, soleus, posterior tibialis*

- 16. 'ARM CRACKER'
  Stretched: *Anterior tibialis, ankle and foot flexors*
  Pressed: *Hamstrings, gastrocnemius*

- 17. FLEXING & STRETCHING THE LEG
  Stretched: *Gastrocnemius, soleus (leg extended); hamstrings, gluteus (leg flexed)*

HEALING BENEFITS

- *Powerfully loosening and stimulating on the knee joint.*

CAUTION!

This technique must not be practised on those who have had any kind of knee or hip surgery.

65

18 PRESSING FOOT TO THIGH

Grasp your partner's right foot. Place your right foot diagonally with the arch across the back of her thigh. Lean back, pulling the leg towards you to generate a strong, sustained pressure on her hamstrings. Release the pressure, move the foot to a lower position and pull. Repeat several times to cover the whole of the thigh.

HEALING BENEFITS

• *Treats sports injuries to the hamstrings, lower back, hip pain and some forms of sciatica.*

19 'TUG OF WAR'

From the same position as the previous technique, push your partner's left knee forwards while, at the same time, repositioning your toes so that they are grasping the lower edge of her pelvic girdle.

Pressing in with your foot, lean back strongly to straighten her leg and lift her hip onto your toes.

HEALING BENEFITS

• *Very effective for lower back and sciatic pain.*

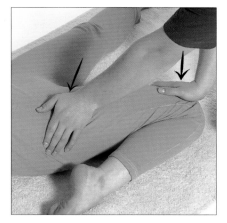

20   PRESSING THE TURNED-IN LEG

If your partner is flexible enough, place her leg with the thigh turned in and the lower leg everted. If not, use your own knee to support her knee. Single or butterfly press the outer margin of the thigh.

HEALING BENEFITS

• *Very effective in the treatment of sciatica and it also improves mobility of the knees.*

21   PRESSING THE LEANING LEG

HEALING BENEFITS

• *Loosens the hip joint to give enhanced flexibility and stimulates energy flow in the outer channels.*
• *Aids mobility of the spine and helps to relieve lower back pain.*

Reposition your partner's leg so that it now leans against her straight one. Palmar press the exposed thigh area several times. Finish by placing one hand over the hip joint and the other on the knee, and pressing very firmly. Hold for at least ten seconds.

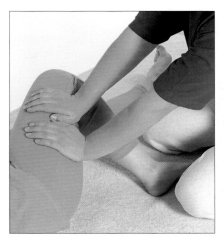

HEALING BENEFITS

• *Very effective for lower back and sciatic pain.*

MUSCLES STRETCHED & PRESSED

• 18. PRESSING FOOT TO THIGH
Pressed: *Hamstrings*

• 19. 'TUG OF WAR'
Pressed: *Hamstrings, gracilis*
Stretched: *Anterior tibialis, quadriceps*

• 20. PRESSING THE TURNED-IN LEG
Stretched: *Quadriceps, sartorius*
Pressed: *Vastus lateralis, vastus intermedius, rectus femoris*

• 21. PRESSING THE LEANING LEG
Pressed: *Vastus lateralis, biceps femoris, tensor fasciae latae*

Place your partner's right leg over her left and locate the foot in position by placing the arch of your right foot lightly across her toes.

Tuck your left hand under her right upper hip while pushing her right knee towards the mat on her left side. Establish a to-and-fro rocking movement aiming to get the knee closer to the floor with each rock.

HEALING BENEFITS

• *Aids lower back and hip flexibility; good for those who suffer from lower back pain.*

23 SHOULDER TO OPPOSITE KNEE SPINAL TWIST

As you finish the previous technique, hold your partner's right knee down in its most extreme position, place your left hand on the front of her right shoulder and press smoothly and firmly. Hold for at least ten seconds.

HEALING BENEFITS

- *Treats lumbar and hip pain.*
- *Increases spinal mobility.*

CAUTION!

When pressing your partner's shoulder down, this must be done carefully with full awareness of your partner's reactions.

24 STRETCHING THE CROSSED LEG HORIZONTALLY

Move to the other side of your partner and extend her right leg across her left hip, holding her right ankle and pressing down on her right hip. Stretch the leg by pushing it towards her head with your knee. Keep the leg straight and only stretch as far as is comfortable.

HEALING BENEFITS

- *Improves hip flexibility, eases tension in the buttocks and hamstrings.*
- *Treats lower back pain and sciatica.*

MUSCLES STRETCHED & PRESSED

- **22. ROCKING THE HIP**
  Stretched: *Quadratus lumborum, piriformis*
  Pressed: *Vastus lateralis, biceps femoris, tensor fasciae latae*

- **23. SHOULDER TO OPPOSITE KNEE SPINAL TWIST**
  Stretched: *Quadratus lumborum, piriformis*
  Pressed: *Vastus lateralis, rectus femoris, biceps femoris*

- **24. STRETCHING THE CROSSED LEG HORIZONTALLY**
  Stretched: *Gastrocnemius, biceps femoris, piriformis, gluteus maximus, soleus*
  Pressed: *Gluteus maximus*

25 PRESSING IN THE SPLITS POSITION

Spread your partner's legs apart as far as is comfortable and hold them in this position with your feet. Palmar and thumb press the inner Sen channels in her lower leg and the thigh.

26 SWINGING THE LEG IN THE SPLITS POSITION

Support the top of your partner's thigh *(right)* with your right hand and grasp her heel with the other. Swing her leg out to the side as far as is comfortable for her. Then swing backwards and forwards several times.

27   HALF LOTUS PRESS

Touch Method One (below) Lift your partner's leg into a Half Lotus position with her ankle lying above her left knee. Should she be very stiff, you will need to support her flexed leg across your knee. With your right hand holding down her left thigh, press up and down the inner energy Sen of her flexed leg with a rocking motion.

Touch Method Two (right) Repeat, using the thumb walking technique.

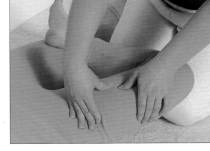

HEALING BENEFITS

• *Aids flexibility of the ankles, knees and hips.*
  • *Provides intense stimulation of the inner Sen to help remove energy blocks.*

28   HALF LOTUS HIP ROCK

With your partner still in the Half Lotus position, lift her straightened left leg across your right thigh. Holding the foot and knee of her flexed right leg, rock the knee to and fro sideways.

HEALING BENEFITS

• *Improves knee and hip mobility and treats lower lumbar, sacral and sciatic pain.*

MUSCLES STRETCHED & PRESSED

• 25. PRESSING IN THE SPLITS POSITION
  Stretched: *Adductors, gracilis, gastrocnemius, hamstrings*
  Pressed: *All the stretched muscles*

• 26. SWINGING THE LEG IN THE SPLITS POSITION
  Stretched: *Adductors, gracilis, gastrocnemius, hamstrings*
  Pressed: *All the stretched muscles*

• 27. HALF LOTUS PRESS
  Stretched: *Adductors, gracilis*
  Pressed: *Adductors, gracilis*

• 28. HALF LOTUS HIP ROCK
  Stretched: *Hamstrings (straight leg), gluteus maximus (flexed leg)*

29   HALF LOTUS BACK ROCK & ROLL

HEALING BENEFITS

• *Eases back pain and improves back and hip mobility.*

Still in the Half Lotus, hold your partner's right heel and push her right leg forward over her head while stabilizing her buttocks with your other hand. Establish a to-and-fro rocking action.

30   VERTICAL HALF LOTUS THIGH PRESS

Maintaining the Half Lotus, lift your partner's straightened left leg into a vertical position, supporting her ankle against your shoulder. Hold the ankle of her other foot and palmar press the exposed thigh from knee to buttock keeping your arm straight and rocking forward with each press.

HEALING BENEFITS

• *Treats lower back pain and sciatica and improves mobility in the hip and knee.*

31 CORKSCREW

With your partner's right leg still firmly in the Half Lotus, hold her left leg vertically. Move forward and step over her flexed right leg with your left one. Place your left foot so that your toes are under her armpit and keep your knees slightly flexed. Tuck your right leg against the outer margin of her vertical leg and use it to support her leg. By gradually straightening your left leg you will exert a backward pressure on her flexed leg and this will generate a twisting action on the hips and lower back. Knead the sole and the heel of her left foot with your right elbow.

CAUTION!

Be careful not to overdo the twisting action. If your partner is very stiff, stand further back with your right leg and only raise and push her straight leg as far as it will comfortably go without twisting the hips with your other leg. Do not use on elderly people.

MUSCLES STRETCHED & PRESSED

- 29. HALF LOTUS BACK ROCK & ROLL
  Stretched: *Hamstrings (straight leg); adductors, gracilis (flexed leg)*

- 30. VERTICAL HALF LOTUS THIGH PRESS
  Stretched: *Gluteus maximus (bent leg); soleus, gastrocnemius, hamstrings (straight leg)*

- 31. CORKSCREW
  Stretched: *Adductors, vastus medialis, gracilis (flexed leg), gastrocnemius, soleus, hamstrings (straight leg)*

HEALING BENEFITS

- *Treats lumbago and sciatica.*
- *Increases hip and lower back flexibility.*

32   RAISED FOOT LEG STRETCH

Grasp your partner's right heel and lift her leg while pressing down on the top of her thigh with your other hand. As you lift, simultaneously press down on the sole of her foot with your forearm.

HEALING BENEFITS

• *Helps myofascial release in the calf muscles to ease pain and tension.*

33   VERTICAL LEG STRETCH

Raise your partner's right leg to as near vertical as is comfortable and support her heel or ankle against the front of your shoulder. Keep her leg straight with your other hand across her knee. Kneel very lightly across her left thigh to hold it down. Gently push the leg forward several times, each time slightly increasing the stretch.

HEALING BENEFITS

• *Treats and relaxes tense or spasming calf and hamstring muscles resulting from sports injuries, sciatica and back pain.*

34 SEESAW LEG STRETCH

Sit very lightly on your partner's right groin facing her feet. Grasp her right foot with both hands and lift the leg towards you.

HEALING BENEFITS

• *Relieves knee ligament pain and treats spasming or injured calf and hamstring muscles.*

CAUTION!

If your partner is very stiff, care must be taken not to lift the leg too far. Do not even attempt this technique with an elderly partner.

CAUTION!

Take care when kneeling along the top of your partner's thigh.

To increase the stretch down the back of her leg, pull the front of the foot gently downwards and rock to and fro. Use small rotary movements to rotate the hip joint.

MUSCLES STRETCHED & PRESSED

• 32. RAISED FOOT LEG STRETCH
  Stretched: *Hamstrings, peroneus longus, gastrocnemius, soleus*

• 33. VERTICAL LEG STRETCH
  Stretched: *Hamstrings, gastrocnemius, soleus, peroneus longus (foot pressed down)*

• 34. SEESAW LEG STRETCH
  Stretched: *Gastrocnemius, hamstrings*
  Pressed: *Quadriceps*

75

BOTH LEGS & BACK

The aim of this lesson is to stimulate energy flow between the trunk and legs. A healthy backbone needs to bend and rotate in many directions. Pain in the lumbar area is very common and can be caused not only by sports injuries, but by poor posture. Acute pain can be triggered by sudden twisting of the waist or lifting heavy loads. Many of the techniques featured here provide powerful muscle stretches which can correct postural imbalances and relax spasming muscles, thereby relieving back pain.

Sen channels on the legs and back

• ③ – Chinese Bladder meridian. This starts between the Achilles tendon and the outer ankle bone and runs up the back of the leg approximately on the midline to the lower border of the buttocks.

• ③ – Thai bodywork uses two back Sen channels along the Chinese Bladder meridian. There are two lines on each side of the spine. The inner one is about two finger-widths and the outer one four finger-widths from the midline of the spine.

ABOVE: *Shown are the third outer Sen channel on each leg and the two Sen on either side of the spine, the health of which depends on the free flow of energy through them.*

1   PRESSING THE INNER FEET & LEGS

Repeat the first technique in Lesson Two *(see page 56)*. Re-establishing contact with the feet encourages a sense of body and mind integration and general well-being. As the inner Sen start on the feet and legs, pressing the inner legs stimulates energy flow between the legs and trunk.

MUSCLES STRETCHED & PRESSED

- 1. PRESSING THE INNER FEET & LEGS
  Stretched: *Adductors*

- 2. LEG BLOOD STOP
  Pressed: *Adductors*

2   LEG BLOOD STOP

Your partner should be lying supine in a totally relaxed position with his legs slightly apart. Kneel and palm up both his thighs until your palms reach the groin area. Press down and adjust your hands until you feel his blood pulsing through the femoral arteries beneath the heels of your palms.

Now lift your body by straightening your legs or arching your buttocks. This will focus your weight on your palms, thus increasing pressure on his arteries to restrict the flow of blood through them. Hold for thirty to fifty seconds.

HEALING BENEFITS

- *When blood flow into the legs is interrupted, the entire circulation including lymphatic drainage is reduced or completely stopped. The swift rush of blood into the legs is accompanied by a sudden spread of warmth down to the feet as full circulation is restored. After this treatment the legs feel very light.*

CAUTION!

Do not attempt to carry out this technique on those with any kind of circulatory problem such as varicose veins, high blood pressure or heart disease.

3   BOW & ARROW SPINAL TWIST

Tuck your right heel behind your partner's left flexed knee and grasp and pull his left forearm towards you *(below)*, keeping his left leg firmly located on the mat. Now lean across and grasp under his left shoulder *(inset right)* with both hands and pull it up towards you.

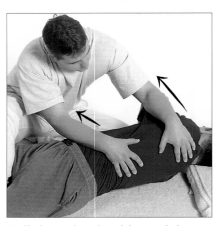

Pull along the shoulder and down your partner's side with alternate hand movements which should be kept slow and rhythmical.

CAUTION!

Do not use on those who have had surgery on the lower back.

4   ROTATING THE HIPS

Lift your partner's flexed legs so that his knees are directly over his abdomen. Your legs should be astride his ankles with your hands just below his knees. Starting with just a small amplitude rotation of the knees, gradually increase. Keep both knees together. Rotate about fifteen times in each direction.

HEALING BENEFITS

• *Has a soothing effect on those who experience stiffness in the hip region, sciatica and lower back pain. In addition to the rotation imposed on the hip joint, a twisting action on the lumbar vertebral also occurs and this relaxes muscles in the hip.*

5 SHAKING THE LEGS

Grasp your partner's ankles, lean back slightly to create traction and shake his legs up and down rapidly with a small-amplitude movement. Shake the legs ten to twenty times.

HEALING BENEFITS (5 & 6)

• *Essential for those suffering from lower back pain and sciatica. These techniques can also be used on those who suffer from varicose veins.*

6 SWINGING THE LEGS

Now hold your partner's legs at the ankles and swing from side to side at least fifteen times. Start with small, slow swings that gradually get bigger and faster.

MUSCLES STRETCHED & PRESSED

• 3. BOW & ARROW SPINAL TWIST
Stretched: *Quadratus lumborum, rhomboideus major and minor, levator scapulae, trapezius, erector spinae, iliacus, psoas major*

• 4. ROTATING THE HIPS
Stretched: *Gluteus maximus, quadriceps (slight stretch), quadratus lumborum*

7 ROCKING & ROLLING THE BACK

Use your right hand to hold your partner's heels so that both his legs are straight. Push his feet forward over his head using your other hand to help lift his buttocks. Determine how far he can comfortably roll back and then proceed to rock and roll to-and-fro up to this limit. This requires a very smooth and controlled rocking action from you.

CAUTION!

Care must be taken not to over-stretch anyone to whom you are giving massage for the first time.

HEALING BENEFITS

• *Helps to ease middle and upper back pain.*

8 THE PLOUGH

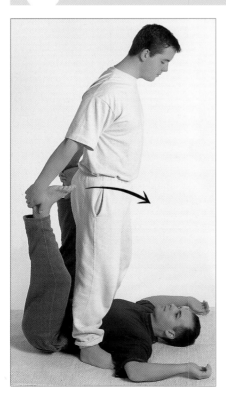

Spread your partner's legs out into an open 'V' and step through them to adopt a new position astride his

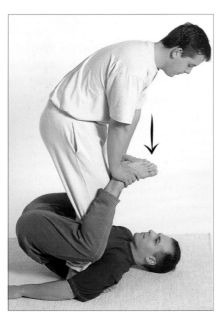

body with your feet tucked under his armpits. Bend your knees slightly towards the mid-line, increase the 'V' angle between his legs and draw them around your knees. Press his feet together and then press lightly downwards. Hold for a few seconds, then open his legs again, draw them back around your legs and push the feet forward and down a little further in the direction of his head. In a very flexible person the feet will touch the floor. Repeat this until you find the most extreme position that is comfortable for him. Hold the position for at least ten seconds.

9   KNEEING THE BACKS OF THE THIGHS

As your partner is released from the previous position, retain your hold on his feet and step back through his legs again. Hold his feet so that his legs are slightly bent. Using your body weight, press both knees simultaneously into the backs of his thighs whilst, at the same time, pushing his feet forward. Press progressively along the entire length of his thighs.

HEALING BENEFITS

• *This simple technique is good for sufferers of sciatica and those who experience problems with their hamstring muscles.*

CAUTION!

• *Do not use this exercise on the elderly and wait for at least two hours if your partner has eaten a large meal.*

MUSCLES STRETCHED & PRESSED

• 7. ROCKING & ROLLING
   THE BACK
   Stretched: *Erector spinae, gastrocnemius*

• 8. THE PLOUGH
   Stretched: *Adductors, soleus, hamstrings, gluteus maximus, erector spinae*

• 9. KNEEING THE BACKS OF
   THE THIGHS
   Stretched: *Erector spinae, gluteus maximus*
   Pressed: *Hamstrings, lower part of gluteus maximus*

HEALING BENEFITS

• *Aids mobility of the hip joints and counters pain in the pelvic region and lower back.*

81

10 KNEEING THE BUTTOCKS

Lift your partner's buttocks off the
mat and support with both hands
while you knead them deeply with
circular movements of your knees.

HEALING BENEFITS

• *Treats sciatic pain.*

11 SHINNING THE THIGHS

Good balance is required for the
correct execution of this technique.
Bend your partner's right leg into a
right angle so that his thigh is lying
against his abdomen. Hold the
other leg outwards and then lean
your left knee inwards so that your
shin presses against his thigh. Shin
progressively along the entire
length of his thigh with a
to-and-fro rocking motion
between each shin press.

HEALING BENEFITS

• *Another excellent treatment for
sciatica; also very effective for
myofascial release around the
hamstrings, particularly for those
who do a great deal of sport.*

12   THE HALF BRIDGE

Press your partner's knees down towards his abdomen and, with your feet slightly apart, bend your knees forward against the arches of his feet.

Grasp his knees between your interlocked hands. Lean back with your full body weight, at the same time bending your legs until they form a 90° angle. Your partner's buttocks will be raised from the mat and, at the most extreme position (below), only his head, shoulders and arms will still remain on the mat. Hold for at least fifteen seconds, giving his back a big stretch.

HEALING BENEFITS

- *Increases blood flow to the head and neck to give your partner an alert and lively feeling.*
- *Eases lower back pain.*

CAUTION!

Do not use this technique on those with cardiac problems and high blood pressure.

MUSCLES STRETCHED & PRESSED

- 10. KNEEING THE BUTTOCKS
  Stretched: *Erector spinae, Gluteus maximus*
  Pressed: *Gluteus maximus*

- 11. SHINNING THE THIGHS
  Stretched: *Gluteus maximus*
  Pressed: *Hamstrings*

- 12. THE HALF BRIDGE
  Stretched: *Quadriceps, rectus abdominis, erector spinae*

Kneeling, push your partner's legs forward until his buttocks lift and slide your knees and thighs under them. When you are in position, grasp your hands around his legs just above knee level and, leaning backwards, hug his legs against you to give his back a good stretch. This is a safe and gentle back stretch compared with the Half Bridge.

HEALING BENEFITS

• *Treats tension and pain in the lower back.*

14 LIFTING HEAD TO STRAIGHT KNEES

Align your partner's legs firmly against the front of your own and lean forward to grasp each arm around the wrist. Lean your weight backwards and pull his upper body forwards and upwards.

Hold the extreme position for up to ten seconds and then gently lower his upper body onto the mat. Repeat this exercise twice and maintain a slow, steady rhythm throughout.

HEALING BENEFITS (14 & 15)

• *Improves shoulder and hip mobility. All the stretched muscles are relaxed.*
• *Can ease sciatic pain.*

MUSCLES STRETCHED & PRESSED

• 13. INTIMATE BACK STRETCH
Stretched: *Erector spinae (lower back), hamstrings*

• 14. LIFTING HEAD TO STRAIGHT KNEES
Stretched: *Teres major & minor, biceps, latissimus dorsi, trapezius, rhomboideus, erector spinae, hamstrings*

• 15. LIFTING HEAD TO CROSSED KNEES
Stretched: *Teres major & minor, rhomboideus, biceps, trapezius, erector spinae, gluteus maximus, latissimus dorsi*

15 LIFTING HEAD TO CROSSED KNEES

As you finish the previous exercise, flex your partner's legs at the knees and cross his ankles, adjusting their position so that the side of each ankle rests against the front of your shins just below your knees. Now grasp his wrists and raise his upper body towards you, just as you did in the last technique. Hold for at least ten seconds and then repeat.

CAUTION!

Good flexibility when the legs are straight is not necessarily an accurate guide to your partner's flexibility when his legs are crossed. Some people have very restricted lateral movement in their hips and/or ankles but good mobility in the forward/backward direction.

Lesson Four

CHEST & ABDOMEN

The techniques demonstrated in Lesson Four stimulate the energies of the internal organs. Deep and thorough abdominal massage boosts the immune system. Always allow three hours after a meal before working the abdomen.

Deciding on what degree of pressure is just right for a particular individual can be difficult. People vary enormously in their ability to tolerate pressure. In Western cultures people are unused to having their abdomens deeply massaged. Thai massage techniques for the abdomen are deeply penetrating. Be attentive to your partner's facial expressions and body reactions, and always obtain verbal confirmation that the pressure exerted is tolerable.

Sen channels on the abdomen

There are nine pressure areas or zones in the abdomen, with the navel in the centre. Start in the lower right section and always press around the abdomen in a clockwise direction.

There are two main techniques. Firstly, thumb walk the lines on the diagram. Start at zone ① and thumb walk all around the edge to zone ⑨. You can then vary this pattern by going ① – ⑤ – ① – ⑤ – ⑨ – ⑤ – ⑨ and then ① – ⑨.

Secondly, double palm press zones ① – ⑤ on the right side and then move to the left side and press zones ⑥ – ⑨.

ABOVE: *These are the nine pressure points on the abdomen, which must be thoroughly pressed if energy balance in the internal organs is to be achieved.*

1   PRESSING THE CHEST, SHOULDERS & ARMS

With your arms straight, palm your partner's upper pectoral region using a slow, rocking movement of your body to generate pressure.

Take care not to press this area too hard. If your partner is a man, you can palm the entire pectoral area. Now extend the palming down the

arms to the hands, keeping the pressure even throughout. Palm back up the arms and repeat the palming of the pectorals.

HEALING BENEFITS

• *Techniques 1, 2 and 3 are designed to tone the internal organs, particularly the lungs, and benefit asthma/bronchitis sufferers.*
• *Palming the arms contributes to the overall energy balance within the body.*

2   PRESSING THE CHEST

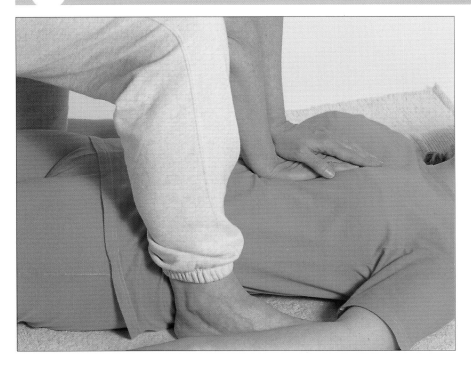

Maintaining your position, use both hands as shown to palm press down the midline of your partner's chest on the breastbone. Press with a to-and-fro pushing movement to create a rocking effect and, with a female partner, always restrict your pressing to these areas.

MUSCLES STRETCHED & PRESSED

• 1. PRESSING THE CHEST, SHOULDERS & ARMS
Pressed: *Pectorals, deltoids, biceps, wrist extensors*

3   PRESSING BETWEEN THE RIBS (INTERCOSTAL MUSCLES)

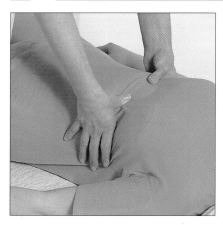

Touch Method One Thumb press the intercostal spaces between your partner's ribs simultaneously outwards from the sternum. Start with both thumbs either side of the sternum just below the collar bone and progress downwards. If you have a female partner, be prepared to press some of the intercostal spaces in the centre only. Also, be sensitive to those for whom the rib spaces are major tickling spots!

Touch Method Two Now use your three middle fingers of both hands to press across the ribs with a small circular motion. Again, progress downwards, observing the same precautions as for the intercostal pressing.

4   THUMB WALKING THE ABDOMEN

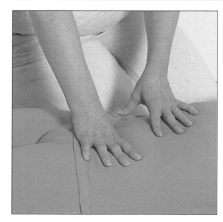

HEALING BENEFITS

• *Encourages the smooth flow of energy through the abdominal Sen to relax the abdominal muscles.*

Kneeling on your partner's right, use the thumb walking technique and start just above her groin on the right side in zone ①. Thumb walk slowly, rhythmically and deeply without causing pain to the right side across the abdomen just below the rib line, and down the left side to just above the pubic bone from zone ① to zone ⑨.

Repeat this circuit several times and then thumb down the mid-line a few times. You can vary this pattern by thumbing clockwise around the two triangular areas shown on page 86.

5 PALM PRESSING THE ABDOMEN

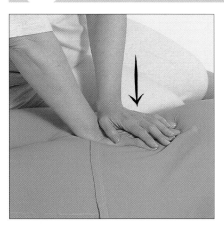

Imagine your partner's abdomen divided into nine equal zones with the navel in the centre. Begin in zone ①. As she exhales, press with the heels of both hands aiming towards the navel and gradually and carefully increase the pressure. Hold for up to two minutes.

Ask her to take a deep breath as you release the pressure. Repeat for zones ② to ⑤. Move to her left and continue on zones ⑥ to ⑨.

HEALING BENEFITS (5 & 6)

• *Regular massage using Exercises 5 and 6 aids digestion, relieves heartburn and constipation, also the heaviness experienced in the lower abdomen during the pre-menstrual period.*

6 PRESSING FEET TO STOMACH

Sit between your partner's legs, hold her hands and carefully place the balls of your feet side by side on the upper abdomen. Press alternately with care to cover the whole abdomen.

MUSCLES STRETCHED & PRESSED

• 3. PRESSING BETWEEN THE RIBS
Pressed: *Intercostals*

• 4. THUMB WALKING THE ABDOMEN
Pressed: *All abdominals*

• 5. PALM PRESSING THE ABDOMEN
Pressed: *All abdominals*

• 6. PRESSING FEET TO STOMACH
Pressed: *All abdominals*

Lesson Five

ARMS, HANDS, NECK & FACE

Arms feed vital energy into the body's organ systems and need thorough treatment to ensure smooth energy flow. Shoulders store tension which causes neck pain and headaches. Stretching the shoulders and neck relieves the tension, while pressure on the head energizes and calms the mind.

Sen channels on the arms

Ⓐ Inner Sen channels

- ① – Starts behind the thumb under the wrist and ends on deltoid muscle.
- ② – Starts on the underside of the wrist in the midline and passes between radius and ulna bones towards the armpit, where it ends.
- ③ – Starts on the underside of the wrist behind the little finger and ends in the armpit.

Ⓑ Outer Sen Channels

- ① – Starts on the wrist crease behind the thumb and passes along the edge of the radius to the outer elbow and up to the front of the shoulder.
- ② – Starts on the middle of the wrist crease and passes between the radius and ulna and then over the humerus to the deltoid muscle.
- ③ – Starts on the wrist crease behind the little finger and passes up to the back of the armpit.

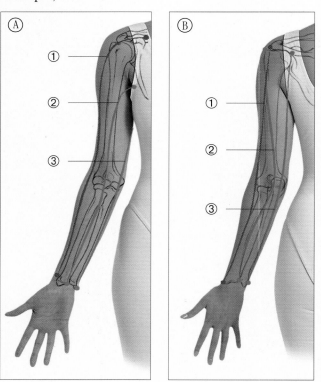

The Inner Sen channels (left) are: ① – Chinese Lung meridian, ② – Chinese Pericardium meridian, ③ – Chinese Heart meridian. The Outer Sen channels (right) are: ① – Chinese Large Intestine meridian, ② – Chinese Sanjiao meridian, ③ – Chinese Small Intestine meridian.

1 PRESSING THE INNER ARM

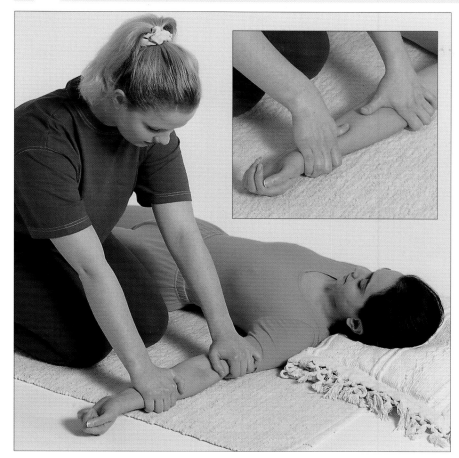

Touch Method One: Palmar Pressing Place your partner's arm at right angles to her body with the palm uppermost. Palm the inner Sen *(far left)* keeping your arms straight and bring your body weight forward to create slow, deep pressure. Do this several times, both up and down the Sen.

Touch Method Two: Thumb Pressing Thumb the three Sen channels *(see inset)* using the thumb walking technique. Maintain a slow, steady rhythm throughout and cover the channels, working up and down at least three times.

2 PRESSING THE OUTER ARM

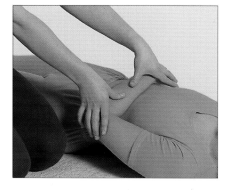

Touch Method One Lift your partner's arm and place it palm downwards across her chest. This exposes the outer Sen channels which can now be palmed and thumbed using exactly the same techniques as those used on the inner Sen channels.

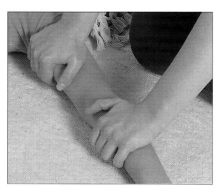

Touch Method Two Place your partner's arm palm downwards on the mat. Change your kneeling position to one behind her arm. Palm and thumb the outer Sen channels again.

HEALING BENEFITS

• *Relieves pain and stiffness in wrists, elbows and upper arms. Balances Sen energies.*

MUSCLES STRETCHED & PRESSED

• 1. PRESSING THE INNER ARM
Pressed: *Biceps, wrist flexors*

• 2. PRESSING THE OUTER ARM
Pressed: *Deltoids, wrist extensors*

3   FOOT TO ARMPIT STRETCH

Hold your partner's left hand and carefully place your foot in her armpit. Lean back to create a strong pull against the pressure of your foot. Hold for ten seconds.

HEALING BENEFITS

• *Stretches the shoulder muscles to relieve tension.*

4   STRETCHING THE ARM IN THE TRIANGLE POSITION

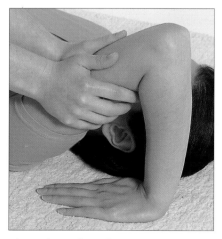

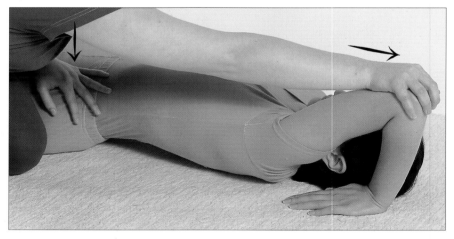

Place the palm of your partner's left hand on the mat with her fingers directed towards her shoulder. Palm the exposed area from elbow to armpit and back again.

Now place your left hand on the upper thigh and your right hand on her elbow. Press down with both hands simultaneously to create a strong stretch across the trunk between arm and thigh.

HEALING BENEFITS

• *Provides a rare treat for the triceps muscles which are the recipient of the palming.*
• *Eases pain and improves mobility in the shoulders.*

5 PRESSING THE TENDONS OF THE UPPER HAND

Starting from the wrist each time, thumb press along and across each of the five main tendons on the back of your partner's hand.

HEALING BENEFITS

• *Strengthens the hands and eases stiffness.*

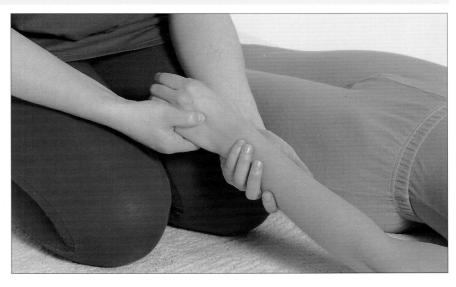

6 ROTATING, PRESSING & PULLING THE FINGERS

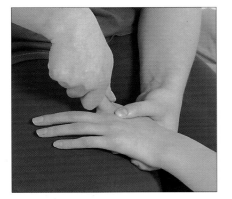

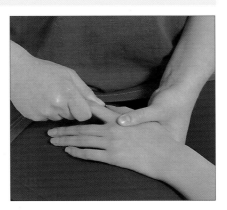

MUSCLES STRETCHED & PRESSED

• 3. FOOT TO ARMPIT STRETCH
Pressed: *Deltoid, rhomboideus, trapezius, infraspinatus, supraspinatus*

• 4. STRETCHING THE ARM IN THE TRIANGLE POSITION
Stretched: *Triceps, latissimus dorsi, pectoralis major, wrist flexors*
Pressed: *Triceps*

Touch Method One Holding each finger in turn at the finger-tips, rotate the fingers several times in both directions.

Touch Method Two Now squeeze up and down each finger using your index finger and thumb. Squeeze first along the top and underside of each finger, followed by lateral squeezing.

HEALING BENEFITS

• *Strengthens the fingers and guards against osteo-arthritis.*

Touch Method Three Pull each finger in turn and use a strong, sliding action to create the necessary extension. Do not be deterred by any cracking sounds that you hear when sharply extending the finger joints as these are not harmful.

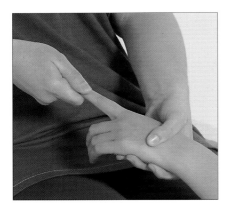

7　KNEE TO HAND PRESSING

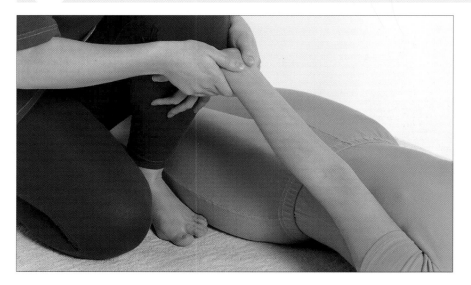

Press your partner's left palm against your knee or upper shin to flex the wrist and fingers backwards. Thumb press the heel of the palm and the wrist.

HEALING BENEFITS

• *Relieves carpal tunnel syndrome, numbness and stiffness.*

8　INTERLOCKED HAND PRESSING

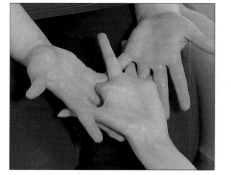

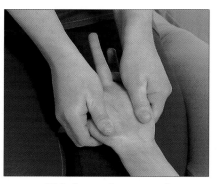

With your partner's palm uppermost, interlock your fingers with those of your partner as follows:
• The fourth finger between fingers five and four.

• Your fifth finger between fingers four and three.
• Your right-hand fifth finger between fingers three and two.
• Your third and fourth fingers

between index finger and thumb.

Slide your fingers under the back of her hands leaving your thumbs free to press her inside wrist and palm. Turn your hands outwards so the sides of your partner's palms are pulled downwards, leaving them arched and stretched. Press deeply wherever you can.

HEALING BENEFITS

• *Gives a powerful backwards stretch to the hand and digits, and relieves numbness and stiffness.*

9　ROTATING THE WRIST

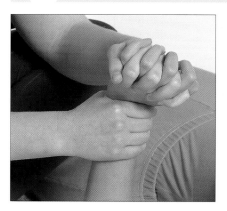

Support your partner's forearm near the wrist and use an interlocked finger grip to rotate her wrist strongly, first one way and then the other.

HEALING BENEFITS

• *Improves overall wrist mobility and relieves numbness of the wrists and hands.*

10 PULLING THE ARMS

Touch Method One: Vertical Arms
Standing behind your partner's shoulders, grasp both her hands and then pull both arms up and down, lifting each shoulder alternately.

MUSCLES STRETCHED & PRESSED

- 7. KNEE TO HAND PRESSING
  Stretched: *Hand flexors*

- 8. INTERLOCKED HAND PRESSING
  Stretched: *Hand flexors*

- 9. ROTATING THE WRIST
  Stretched: *Wrist & hand flexors & extensors*

- 10. PULLING THE ARMS
  Stretched: *Trapezius, deltoids, infraspinatus, rhomboideus, biceps, pectoralis major*

Touch Method Two: Backward Pull
Now step back from your partner and pull both her arms together leaning with your body weight to create the pull.

HEALING BENEFITS

- *Reduces tension in the shoulders and improves mobility of the shoulders.*

11　PRESSING THE SHOULDERS

Kneel behind your partner's head. Press and push the top of her shoulders with both hands, initially sustaining the press for several seconds. Then press and push alternately without holding the presses. Finally, thumb press along the upper border of her collar bone and over the upper regions of the pectoral muscles.

HEALING BENEFITS

• *Helps take tension from the neck and shoulders, and improves shoulder mobility.*

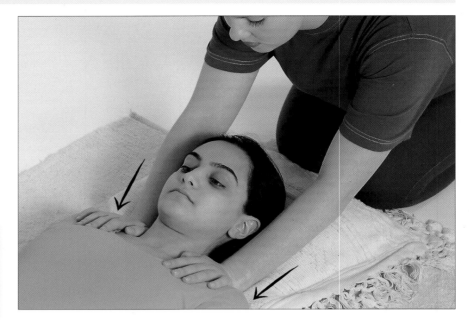

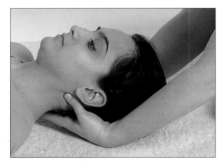

12　PRESSING THE NECK

Support the base of your partner's head with one hand, lifting it slightly forward so that your other hand can press up and down the muscles on one side of her neck. Swap hands to press the other side.

Turn your partner's head to the right so that it rests on the right temple. Press along the full length of the sternocleidomastoid muscle with your left thumb.

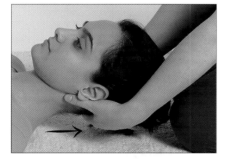

13　STRETCHING THE NECK

Place both hands under your partner's lower neck and pull them towards you to create a mild traction on the neck. Repeat several times. Keeping a slight traction, press with your fingers

into the soft tissue immediately behind the base of the skull. Hold for up to one minute. Allow the weight of the head to generate the pressure.

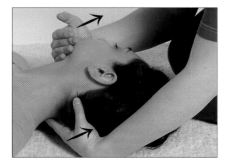

14　PULLING THE TURNED HEAD

Place your right hand under your partner's chin and your left hand under the base of her skull using equal pressure with both hands. Pull her head back very gently and carefully. Hold the pull for at least ten seconds.

HEALING BENEFITS

• *Relaxes the neck muscles, eases headaches and improves mobility of the neck.*

15   MASSAGING THE FACE & HEAD

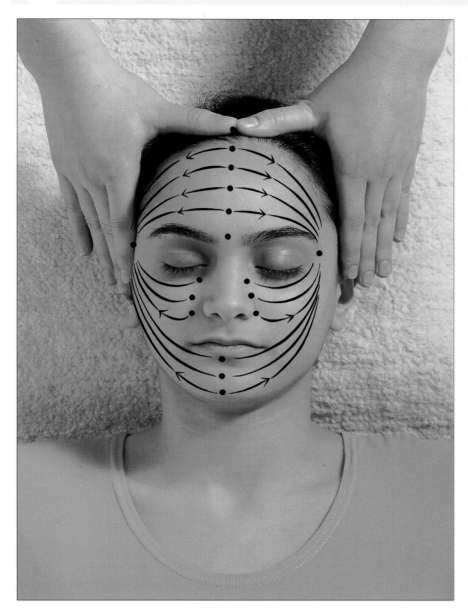

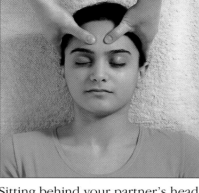

Sitting behind your partner's head, place both thumbs on top of her forehead on the hairline. Press evenly on either side of her face following the directions of the arrows as shown.

HEALING BENEFITS

• *Relaxes the face, eases headaches, calms the mind, relieves nasal congestion, improves hearing and massages the gums.*

16   MASSAGING THE EARS

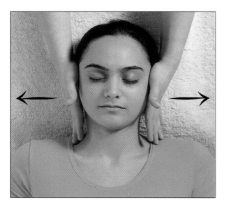

Cup and cover your partner's ears with the palm of your hands to create a suction. Hold for 30 seconds and then release.

HEALING BENEFITS

• *Clears blocked ears.*

MUSCLES STRETCHED & PRESSED

• 11. PRESSING THE SHOULDERS
Pressed: *Trapezius*

• 12. PRESSING THE NECK
Pressed: *Sternocleidomastoid, levator scapulae*

• 14. PULLING THE TURNED HEAD
Stretched: *Sternocleidomastoid, trapezius, erector spinae, levator scapulae*

Lesson Six

LYING ON EITHER SIDE

The techniques featured in this lesson give access to the Sen energy channels in the side position and provide an opportunity to reach muscles that cannot be effectively treated in the other positions. Each side of the body is treated in turn, first with your partner on one side using Exercises 1–23, which are then repeated when he is lying on the other side. If you decide to do only some of the techniques shown, remember to repeat each one on the other side of the body. Refer to Part One Chapter Two (see pages 34–41) for the basic techniques of pressing and manipulation.

Sen channels in the side position

The Sen channels in the legs and back are described and illustrated anatomically in Lessons Two and Seven (see pages 52–53 and 110). In the side position the inside and back of the straight leg exposes the Inner ③ – Chinese Kidney meridian, and the Outer ③ – Chinese Bladder meridian. The kidneys and bladder control water balance in the body as well as treating lower back pain. The bent leg exposes the Outer ② – Gallbladder meridian, and the Outer ③ – Bladder. The energies of the Gallbladder meridian treat leg pain and numbness resulting from sciatica.

ABOVE: *Sen channels accessible in the side position. The Sen channels on the back treat all the internal organs of the body.*

1   PRESSING THE BACK OF THE EXTENDED LEG

Touch Method One: Palmar Pressing (below) Draw your partner's right leg up in front of him so that it forms an angle of about 90° with his body. Keep your arms straight and palm with both hands along the inner Sen of the straight leg using your body weight to generate deep pressure. Palm outwards from the knee and back again several times. Keep a steady rhythm using a slow, to-and-fro rocking movement. Then butterfly palm the entire leg.

Touch Method Two: Thumb Walking (right) Starting on your partner's inside lower leg, thumb walk deeply along the Sen channels.

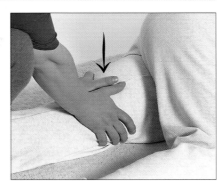

HEALING BENEFITS

• *Pressing the inner Sen channels promotes energy movement through the abdomen and is good for PMT, genital problems and swelling.*

MUSCLES STRETCHED & PRESSED

• 1. PRESSING THE BACK OF THE EXTENDED LEG
Pressed: *Soleus, gastrocnemius, hamstrings, adductor muscles*

• 2. PRESSING THE FLEXED LEG
Pressed: *Gluteus maximus, biceps femoris, tensor fasciae latae, vastus lateralis, ilio-tibial tract*

2   PRESSING THE FLEXED LEG

First, palm the outer Sen channels of your partner's flexed leg. Then thumb walk the Sen energy channels on the lower and the upper leg in turn.

HEALING BENEFITS

• *Stimulates movement of intrinsic energy and helps to release blockages which cause pain and stiffness. Eases and soothes sciatic pain in the legs.*

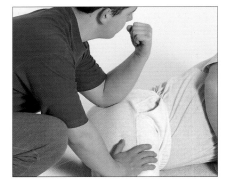

3   PRESSING AROUND THE HIP JOINT

With your partner's right leg still in the flexed position, press deeply with your thumbs and palms around his hip joint. Finally elbow press by leaning in gradually with your body weight to give more pressure.

HEALING BENEFITS

• *Wonderfully effective in the treatment of sciatica.*

4   SIDE SINGLE GRAPE PRESS

Grasp both your partner's ankles and use your right foot to press up and down his thigh. Generate pressure by leaning back and pulling both his legs.

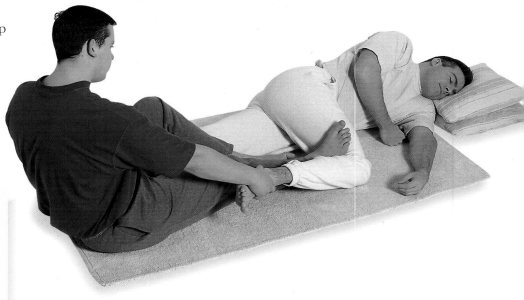

HEALING BENEFITS

• *Eases hip pain.*
• *Encourages relaxation of the hamstring muscles.*

5   SIDE SINGLE GRAPE PRESS & TWISTED VINE

As you complete the previous technique, tuck your foot behind your partner's right knee and cross his right foot over your right shin. Tuck his toes in behind your knee, holding his heel with your right hand. Press up and down his thigh using your left foot.

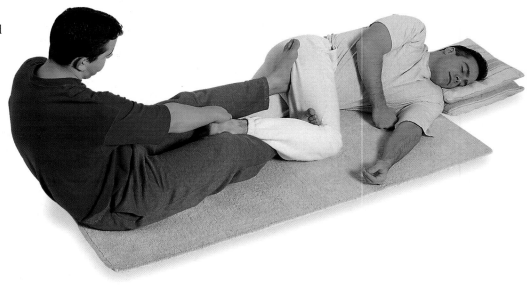

6   SIDE Z-STOP

Follow exactly the same method as used for this technique in the supine position *(see page 60).*

HEALING BENEFITS (4, 5 & 6)

• *Wonderful for troublesome hamstring muscles; sciatic pain felt deeply within the leg also responds well to these treatments.*

• *Leaves the leg suffused with warmth and feeling really light.*

7   FOOT PRESSING THIGHS & CALVES WITH CHAIR

Use a chair to provide you with support as you very carefully step onto the lower part of your partner's flexed legs only, as shown. Without moving the position of your feet on his legs, slowly rock from one foot to the other. Now move your feet to a new position and then repeat.

CAUTION!

Do not attempt this exercise on someone who is lighter than you.

HEALING BENEFITS

• *Relaxes tense and sore muscles and tendons; eases sciatic pain.*

MUSCLES STRETCHED & PRESSED

• 3. PRESSING AROUND THE HIP JOINT
Pressed: *Gluteus maximus, biceps femoris, rectus femoris, tensor fasciae latae*

• 4. SIDE SINGLE GRAPE PRESS
Pressed: *Hamstrings, gluteus maximus, adductors, gracilis*

• 5. SIDE SINGLE GRAPE PRESS & TWISTED VINE
Pressed: *Hamstrings, gluteus maximus, adductors, gracilis*

• 6. SIDE Z-STOP
Stretched: *Quadriceps*
Pressed: *Hamstrings, quadriceps*

• 7. FOOT PRESSING THIGHS & CALVES WITH CHAIR
Pressed: *Gastrocnemius, soleus, hamstrings*

101

8 PRESSING THE BACK IN THE SIDE POSITION

Touch Method One: Palmar Pressing (below) Kneel behind your partner and make sure that his left leg is flexed in front of him to give good support when pressure is applied to his back. Palm press along the two Sen channels to the left of his spine with a rocking movement.

Touch Method Two: Thumb Pressing (inset) Now thumb walk sideways along the same Sen channels on your partner's back.

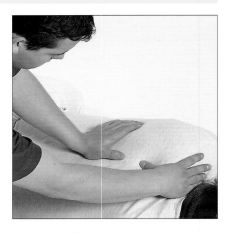

HEALING BENEFITS

• *Pushes the muscles away from the spine, relieving back pain and tension; stimulates energy flow in the Sen benefiting internal organs.*

9 ROTATING THE SHOULDER

Grasp your partner's right shoulder firmly with both your hands. Rotate his shoulder according to his flexibility. Ideally, the rotation should utilize the full range of mobility available to you.

HEALING BENEFITS

• *Restores shoulder mobility.*

10 ROTATING THE SHOULDER WITH ELBOW LEVER

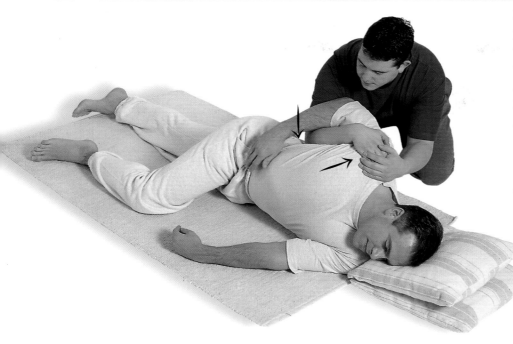

Maintain your grasp on your partner's right shoulder and place your right elbow on his lower back to the right of his spine. Lean forwards so that you can use your elbow as a lever against which you can pull his shoulder as you rotate.

HEALING BENEFITS

- *Improves shoulder mobility and eases shoulder pain.*
- *Relieves pain and tension between the shoulder blades.*

11 PRESSING THE KNEE-SUPPORTED ARM

Extend your partner's right arm and lay it across your left knee. Then palm up and down his arm slowly and firmly several times.

Using your right hand press his axilla while simultaneously pulling his arm back.

HEALING BENEFITS

- *Stretches the pectoral muscles and assists myofascial release in the deltoid and biceps muscles.*

MUSCLES STRETCHED & PRESSED

- 8. PRESSING THE BACK IN THE SIDE POSITION
  Pressed: *Erector spinae, latissimus dorsi, gluteus maximus, quadratus lumborum, trapezius, infraspinatus, rhomboideus major & minor*

- 9. ROTATING THE SHOULDER
  Stretched: *Upper trapezius, pectoralis major, infraspinatus, rhomboideus minor & major*

- 10. ROTATING THE SHOULDER WITH ELBOW LEVER
  Stretched: *Pectoralis major, trapezius, sternocleidomastoid, levator scapulae*

- 11. PRESSING THE KNEE-SUPPORTED ARM
  Pressed: *Biceps, deltoid, flexor muscles of the wrists & hands*

103

12 STRETCHING THE VERTICAL ARM SIDEWAYS

Holding your partner's right hand and wrist, tuck the outside of your lower right leg snugly against your partner's back across the shoulder blades. As you lean back, pull vertically upwards and backwards on his arm, which will be stretched against the outer margin of your right leg. Hold the extreme position for a few seconds and then relax. Repeat several times.

HEALING BENEFITS

• *Improves shoulder mobility.*
• *Eases tension and pain in the elbow region.*

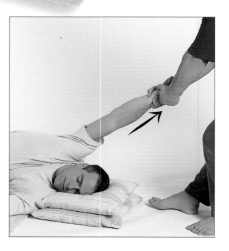

13 PULLING THE ARM IN THE SIDE POSITION

Change your position to pull your partner's arm right back over his head. Relax and then repeat this technique two or three times holding the extreme position in each instance for a few seconds.

HEALING BENEFITS

• *Opens up the shoulder and elbow joints and stimulates the circulation of blood and lymph.*
• *Aids and maintains joint mobility which is especially beneficial for frozen shoulders and tennis elbow.*

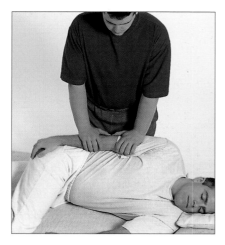

14 PRESSING THE ARM AGAINST THE SIDE

Lay your partner's right arm along his side. Press with both hands along the outer Sen channels of his arm *(see page 92)*. Then thumb walk the Sen channels. Finally, press his wrist and shoulder to give the arm a stretch.

HEALING BENEFITS

• *Stimulates the flow of energy in the Sen channels which contributes to overall energy balance.*

15   STRETCHING THE ARM IN THE TRIANGLE POSITION

Flex your partner's arm at the elbow and place his hand behind his head with his fingers directed towards his shoulder. Palm the exposed upper arm and along the side of his body to the hips. Stretch the side, pressing the elbow and hip.

HEALING BENEFITS

• *Stretches muscles down the side of the body that rarely experience any strong extension.*

MUSCLES STRETCHED & PRESSED

• 12. STRETCHING THE VERTICAL ARM SIDEWAYS
Stretched: *Pectoralis major, trapezius, rhomboideus, teres major, infraspinatus*

• 13. PULLING THE ARM IN THE SIDE POSITION
Stretch: *Latissimus dorsi, teres major, subscapularis*

• 14. PRESSING THE ARM AGAINST THE SIDE
Pressed: *Deltoid, biceps, triceps, hand & wrist extensors*

• 15. STRETCHING THE ARM IN THE TRIANGLE POSITION
Stretched: *Latissimus dorsi, triceps, pectoralis major, hand & wrist flexors, abdominal obliques, quadratus lumborum, teres major*

• 16. SHOULDER TO OPPOSITE KNEE SPINAL TWIST
Stretched: *Abdominal obliques, quadratus lumborum, gluteus maximus, pectoralis major*
Pressed: *Pectoralis major, vastus lateralis, quadriceps*

16   SHOULDER TO OPPOSITE KNEE SPINAL TWIST

With your left hand on your partner's right shoulder and your other hand on his right knee, press down and outwards carefully to generate a good stretch with a twisting action on his spine. Hold the twist for a few seconds.

HEALING BENEFITS

• *Aids spinal flexibility and eases back pain.*

17   KNEE TO KNEE HIP FLEX

Step over your partner's left leg and position yourself with your left leg pressed tightly against his. Hold his right ankle and tuck your right knee behind his while you press down on his right hip. Then push forward and rock with your knee to generate a series of strong hip flexions.

18   STRETCHING THE CROSSED LEG HORIZONTALLY

Straighten your partner's right leg across his left hip, holding his right ankle and pressing down on his right hip. Stretch the leg by pushing it towards his head with your knee. Keep the leg straight and only stretch as far as is comfortable.

19   KNEE PIVOT HIP STRETCH

Place your left knee in the centre of your partner's right buttock. Grasp his right leg and pull it towards you, using your knee as a pivot to help generate a big stretch in the muscles at the front of the hip and thigh. Hold for several seconds, relax slowly and repeat once or twice.

MUSCLES STRETCHED & PRESSED

- 17. KNEE TO KNEE HIP FLEX
  Stretched: *Gluteus maximus, rectus femoris*
  Pressed: *Hamstrings, gluteus maximus*

- 18. STRETCHING THE CROSSED LEG HORIZONTALLY
  Stretched: *Gluteus maximus, piriformis, hamstrings, gastrocnemius, soleus*
  Pressed: *Gluteus maximus, tensor fasciae latae*

- 19. KNEE PIVOT HIP STRETCH
  Stretched: *Quadriceps, gracilis, sartorius, adductors, iliacus, psoas major*
  Pressed: *Gluteus maximus*

  - 20. SIDE BACK BOW
    Stretched: *Quadriceps, psoas major, iliacus, rectus abdominis, pectoralis major*
    Pressed: *Erector spinae, gluteus maximus*

HEALING BENEFITS

- *Eases hip pain and sciatica.*

20   SIDE BACK BOW

Seat yourself on the floor behind your partner with your legs outstretched. Position your feet so that the right one is against his pelvic arch and the left one is across his lumbar region.

Pull your partner's arm and leg towards you, leaning backwards to pull his back against your feet so creating a bow shape through the arm, spine and leg. Hold this pose for a minute or more.

HEALING BENEFITS

- *Improves flexibility of the spine in a backward direction and eases lower back pain.*

21 LATERAL SCISSOR STRETCH

Assume a standing position behind your partner and hold his right arm and leg as shown. Place the arch of your left foot across the top of his right buttock. Maintain only a slight tension on his arm, but pull and lift his leg towards you countering the movement with downward pressure from your foot. Do not press too hard. When you have achieved the appropriate degree of stretch, hold the position for ten seconds.

HEALING BENEFITS

• *Treats hip pain, sciatica and pain down the side of the leg, also lower back pain.*
• *Improves spinal flexibility.*

CAUTION!

For very stiff people, just lifting the leg and arm without using your foot will produce a powerful stretching action. Be careful not to overdo the stretching movements.

22 CROSSED SCISSOR STRETCH

Still holding your partner's right arm, change your position so that you are holding his left leg and move your foot slightly away from his buttock to his extreme lower back. Repeat the stretch as described in the last exercise.

HEALING BENEFITS

As Lateral Scissor Stretch (above).

23 PULLING SPINAL TWIST

Put your right knee into your partner's right buttock while pulling his left arm by leaning backwards with your body weight. Hold for a few seconds, release slowly and repeat once or twice.

HEALING BENEFITS

• *Exercises 23 and 24 stretch the muscles between the shoulders and help to ease frozen shoulders and tennis elbow.*

MUSCLES STRETCHED & PRESSED

• 21 LATERAL SCISSOR STRETCH
Stretched: *Rectus abdominis, iliacus, psoas major, adductors, pectoralis major, sartorius*
Pressed: *Vastus lateralis*

• 22. CROSSED SCISSOR STRETCH
Stretched: As Lateral Scissor Stretch
Pressed: *Vastus lateralis*

• 23. PULLING SPINAL TWIST
Pressed: *Gluteus maximus*
Stretched: *Quadratus lumborum, trapezius, teres major, erector spinae, deltoid, rhomboideus minor & major, infraspinatus, subcapularis*

• 24. LIFTING SPINAL TWIST
Stretched: *Quadratus lumborum, trapezius, teres major, erector spinae, rhomboideus major & minor, infraspinatus, subcapularis*

24 LIFTING SPINAL TWIST

Bend your partner's right leg to form a 90°-angle in front of him, tuck your right foot under the flexed knee and place your left foot on the mat behind him so that the inner margin of your lower leg is firmly against his lower back.

Hold his left wrist as shown and lean backwards using your weight to lift him. Hold for several seconds before lowering him gently to the floor. Repeat twice.

CAUTION!

This exercise must not be practised on anyone who has had spinal surgery such as lumbar fusion or laminectomy, those with osteoporosis or anyone who is much heavier than yourself.

Lesson Seven

PRONE — LYING FACE DOWN

The ultimate energy balance throughout the body can only be achieved by pressing the energy channels on either side of the spine. Energy flow in this area affects all the organ systems and the overall health and well-being of the body. The powerful manipulations demonstrated in this lesson will strengthen the spine and help to treat all kinds of back problems.

Refer to Part One Chapter Two for the basic techniques of pressing and manipulation. Energy flow through the legs and hips relaxes muscle and improves mobility in the lower back as well as all leg and hip joints.

Sen channels on the back

There are two lines on each side of the spine. The inner one is about two finger-widths and the outer line four finger-widths from the midline of the spine. This is ③ – Chinese Bladder meridian.

In Chinese theory the Bladder meridian starts on the eye and ends on the outer edge of the little toe in one continuous energy channel. In Thai bodywork, pressing is done from the feet up to the buttocks. ③ – starts between the ankle bone and the Achilles tendon, then runs up the midline of the back of the leg.

ABOVE: *The Sen channels that run the full length of the spine on both sides have an enormous ability to affect general health and flexibility.*

110

1   STANDING FEET TO FEET PRESS

Balancing your weight on your toes, lean backwards to press your heels into the soles of your partner's feet. Use a gentle to-and-fro rocking motion with your feet. (Note: make sure you have adequate padding beneath his feet for this exercise.)

HEALING BENEFITS

• *Aids flexibility of the foot and improves blood flow as the metatarsal bones are splayed apart.*

MUSCLES STRETCHED & PRESSED

• 1. STANDING FEET TO FEET PRESS
  Pressed: *All intrinsic muscles of the feet*

• 2. PRESSING THE BACK OF THE LEGS & BUTTOCKS
  Pressed: *Gastrocnemius, soleus, hamstrings*

2   PRESSING THE BACK OF THE LEGS & BUTTOCKS

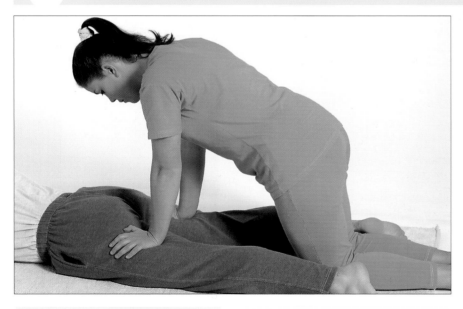

Touch Method One: Palmar and Thumb Pressing Assume a kneeling position and palmar press several times up both your partner's legs simultaneously from the ankles to the lower margin of the buttocks. Now press with your thumbs up the centre Sen channels of the legs *(see page 46)*. Repeat once or twice.

Touch Method Two: Butterfly Pressing Butterfly press up each leg in turn several times.

CAUTION!

Do not use the deep palming or thumbing method on areas with obvious varicose veins.

HEALING BENEFITS

• *Improves blood and lymph circulation and also releases myofascial adhesions.*

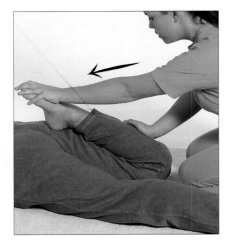

3   PRESSING HEEL TO BUTTOCK

Press your partner's right foot back as far towards the buttocks as is comfortable. At the same time, use the heel of your right palm to press along the Sen which lies just outside the margin of the tibia (shin bone) *(see page 46)*.

HEALING BENEFITS

• *Eases pain and tension in tight and spasming quadriceps; improves ankle and knee mobility.*

4   PRESSING THE THIGH & PULLING THE FOOT

Grasp your partner's foot with both hands and place your right foot across the back of his thigh, close to the knee crease. Pull the lower leg vertically upwards and hold for a few seconds. Move your foot to different positions up the thigh between each vertical pull.

HEALING BENEFITS

• *Eases sciatic pain and relieves pain and tension in the hamstring muscles; aids ankle flexibility and stimulates the Sen channels.*

5   FOOT CRACKER

Still standing, tuck your left foot in snugly behind your partner's right knee and press his foot down towards his buttock.

HEALING BENEFITS

• *Improves mobility of the ankle and knee joints; eases tension and spasming in calves and hamstrings.*

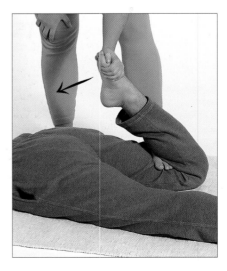

6 STANDING BACKWARD LEG LIFT

Facing your partner's feet, grasp his right ankle and then lift his leg backwards as far as is comfortable.

Now repeat Techniques 3–6 on the other leg.

HEALING BENEFITS

• *Eases lower back and hip pain, and sciatica.*

MUSCLES STRETCHED & PRESSED

• 3. PRESSING HEEL TO BUTTOCK
Stretched: *Tibialis anterior, quadriceps, foot flexors*

• 4. PRESSING THE THIGH & PULLING THE FOOT
Stretched: *Tibialis anterior, foot flexors*
Pressed: *Hamstrings*

• 5. FOOT CRACKER
Stretched: *Tibialis anterior, quadriceps, foot flexors*
Pressed: *Hamstrings, gastrocnemius*

• 6. STANDING BACKWARD LEG LIFT
Stretched: *Iliacus, psoas major, quadriceps, sartorius*

• 7. PRESSING FEET TO BUTTOCK
Stretched: *Anterior tibialis, quadriceps, foot flexors, soleus*

7 PRESSING FEET TO BUTTOCK

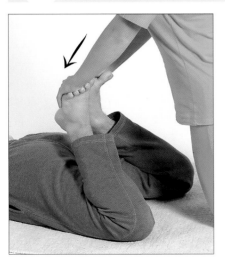

Touch Method One Press both your partner's feet down towards his buttocks and simultaneously pull down on the balls of his feet.
Touch Method Two Cross your partner's legs and press both his feet down to his buttocks. Recross his legs in the opposite way and then repeat.

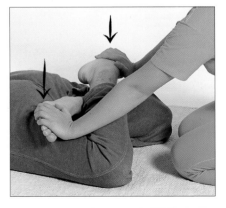

HEALING BENEFITS

Increases mobility of the feet, ankles and knees.

113

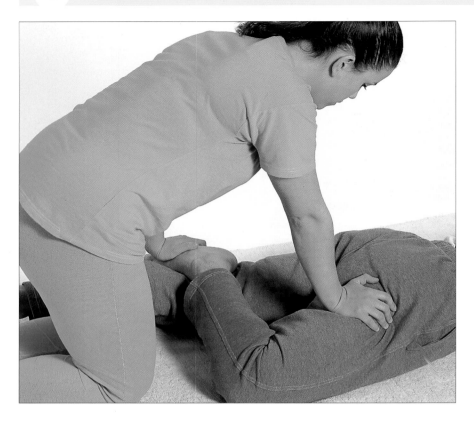

Bend your partner's right leg into the Half Lotus position so that the top of his foot lies across his left thigh just behind the knee crease. Now palm and thumb walk along the outer Sen of the flexed leg *(see page 46)*.

HEALING BENEFITS

• *Improves energy flow through the knees and thighs.*

9   REVERSE HALF LOTUS LEG FLEX

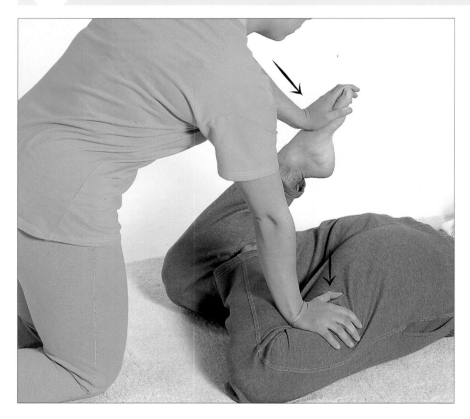

From the same Half Lotus position, grasp your partner's left foot, as shown, and push it down towards his buttock. Then with each push forward simultaneously press his other thigh.

HEALING BENEFITS

• *Stimulates blood flow and lymphatic drainage, and treats painful and spasming hamstrings and sciatica.*

10   REVERSE HALF LOTUS LEG LIFT

Retaining the Half Lotus position of the legs, grasp your partner's left foot with both hands and stand up. Place your right foot carefully across his lower lumbar area and lean in on it *without* using your full body weight as you lift his leg.

CAUTION!

Only with a highy flexible partner will you be able to lift his leg to anywhere near the vertical position.

HEALING BENEFITS

• *Improves flexibility in the hip and knee joints. Treats chronic pain in the ilio-sacral region.*

MUSCLES STRETCHED & PRESSED

• 8. REVERSE HALF LOTUS PRESS
  Pressed: *Hamstrings, vastus lateralis, gastrocnemius, peroneus longus*

• 9. REVERSE HALF LOTUS LEG FLEX
  Stretched: *Tibialis anterior, quadriceps, psoas major, adductors, sartorius*
  Pressed: *Hamstrings, vastus lateralis*

• 10. REVERSE HALF LOTUS LEG LIFT
  Stretched: *Psoas major, quadriceps, iliacus*
  Pressed: *Sacrospinalis*

• 11. KNEE OR HAND TO BUTTOCK/BACK LEG LIFT
  Stretched: *Gracilis, quadriceps*
  Pressed: *Gluteus maximus*

11   KNEE TO BUTTOCK/BACK BACKWARD LEG LIFT

Touch Method One Place your right knee into your partner's right buttock and lift his leg with your hand just above the knee. Use your knee as the pivot against which to lift his leg.

HEALING BENEFITS

• *Helps those who suffer from lumbar and hip pain, and sciatica.*

Touch Method Two With your right hand across your partner's lower lumbar area, lift his right flexed leg against the pressure of your hand.

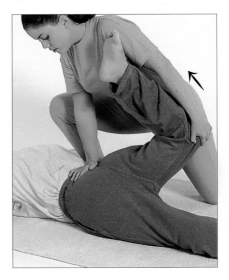

12 FOOT TO BUTTOCK/BACK BACKWARD LEG LIFT

Hold your partner's right foot with both hands and lift his leg. Now place your left foot across his lower lumbar area and lean back to pull the leg against pressure from the foot.

HEALING BENEFITS (12 & 13)

• *Eases tension and pain in front of the thigh, and helps sciatica and lower back pain.*

13 BACKWARD SEESAW LEG LIFT

Sit lightly on your partner's buttocks, taking most of your weight on your feet. Grasp his right knee underneath and, with both hands, lift his leg towards you as far as it will comfortably go without causing pain. Hold for at least ten seconds.

14 INTIMATE CALF & THIGH PRESS

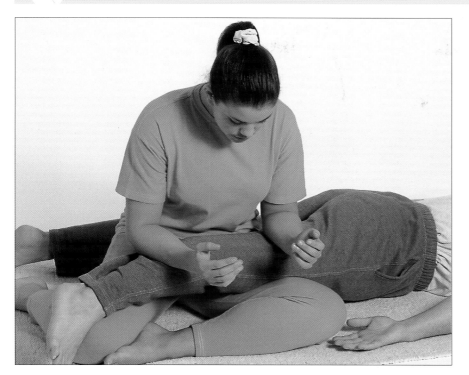

With your partner's right leg over your legs, sit between his thighs. Use your forearms to press along his thigh and calf simultaneously from ankle to buttock. Repeat.

MUSCLES STRETCHED & PRESSED

- 12. FOOT TO BUTTOCK/BACK BACKWARD LEG LIFT
  Stretched: *Iliacus, psoas major, quadriceps*
  Pressed: *Gluteus maximus, sacrospinalis*

- 13. BACKWARD SEESAW LEG LIFT
  Stretched: *Psoas major, iliacus, quadriceps, sartorius*
  Pressed: *Gluteus maximus*

- 14. INTIMATE CALF & THIGH PRESS
  Stretched: *Gluteus, biceps femoris, vastus lateralis*
  Pressed: *Gluteus, biceps femoris, vastus lateralis*

HEALING BENEFITS

- *Treats sciatica and lower back pain and relaxes tense muscles in the leg.*

Then lean in carefully with your elbow and knead the entire buttock area.

Then repeat Exercises 8–14 on the other leg.

Touch Method One: Palmar Pressing (right) Kneel on one leg astride your partner. With your palm heels on either side of his spine and fingers directed outwards, use both hands to palm deeply and very slowly up and down the Sen of his back between the sacro-lumbar and upper thoracic regions, as shown. Keep your arms straight at all times and use your body weight to generate the required pressure. Finish off by palming his arms.

HEALING BENEFITS

• *Stimulates energy flow through the back. Releases tense and fibrotic fascia around back muscles and eases lumbago, sciatica and pain due to slipped disc.*

CAUTION!

Exercise care when carrying out the Cobra exercises. There be should be no trace of jerkiness in the movements as these must, at all times, be smoothly executed for reasons of safety.

Many people will experience real discomfort if you attempt to raise their shoulders more than an inch or so from the mat. This stretch should only be performed on those who are fit and fairly flexible. Do not attempt any of the Cobra techniques on partners heavier than yourself, on the elderly or those with intervertebral disc problems.

16   KNEELING CUSHION COBRA

Kneeling on your partner's thighs, grasp his wrists and ask him to grasp your own wrists. Lean back to use your weight to lift his upper body into a Cobra position. Hold for at least ten seconds.

Modern living provides few opportunities for backward flexion of the spine. To ensure that your partner's spine remains healthy and pain-free, you must do both forward and backward flexions.

Touch Method Two: Thumb Pressing (far left) Use both your thumbs simultaneously to press the first Sen channels of your partner's back, which are located about 2 cm (¾ in) from his spine on both sides.

Touch Method Three (left) This is a variation on Touch Method One where you kneel on the back of the thighs just below the buttocks to palmar or thumb press the whole back.

MUSCLES STRETCHED & PRESSED

- 15. PRESSING THE BACK
  Pressed: *Erector spinae, trapezius, rhomboideus minor & major, quadratus lumborum*

- 16. KNEELING CUSHION COBRA
  Pressed: *Hamstrings*
  Stretched: *Pectoralis major, deltoids, rectus abdominis, psoas, iliacus, serratus anterior*

HEALING BENEFITS (16, 17 & 18)

• *Strong, sustained backward flexion exercises the articulating joints and associated muscles between the vertebrae, particularly the lumbar ones. Spinal mobility and flexibility is improved, tension and pain in the lower back and between the shoulder blades is eased, and increased shoulder mobility results. Energy flow in the Sen channels of the back increases.*

119

Touch Method One Flex your partner's lower legs to 90° so that the soles of his feet are pointing upwards. Sit down carefully on his feet and support your main body weight on your own feet. Palm press the back as described in Exercise 15. Lift his arms back and place his wrists across the tops of your thighs. Bend forward and place your hands under the front of his shoulders and lift them from the mat using your body weight as you lean backwards. Hold for thirty seconds. Then repeat twice.

Touch Method Two This time your partner interlocks his hands behind his head. Repeat the lift, holding his shoulders as in Touch Method One or under the armpits.

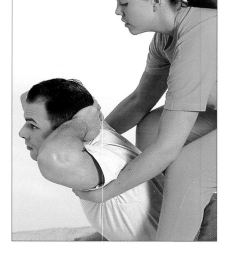

18 STANDING COBRA

Considerable balance is needed to perform this technique correctly. Stand on your partner with one foot placed on each of his thighs. Your toes should be directed to point outwards and the arches of your feet should cover the lower margin of his buttocks. Lean forward, grasp his wrists and he yours simultaneously and, with your arms straight, lean backwards so that your weight is pivoted onto your feet. Now lift him into a Cobra position.

The ability to tolerate backward flexion of the spine varies greatly so much care must be taken on the first lift to determine how far you can go. Each lift should be sustained for up to thirty seconds. Repeat twice.

CAUTION!

Many people will experience real discomfort if you attempt to raise their shoulders more than an inch or so from the mat. This stretch should only be performed on those who are reasonably flexible. Do not attempt any of the Cobra techniques on partners heavier than yourself, on the elderly or those with intervertebral disc problems.

MUSCLES STRETCHED & PRESSED (16, 17 & 18)

Pressed: *Hamstrings*
Stretched: *Pectoralis major; deltoids, teres major, rectus abdominis, psoas major, iliacus, trapezius, infraspinatus, supraspinatus, serratus anterior*

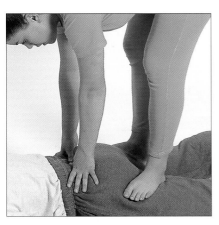

121

19   WHEELBARROW

Grasp your partner's ankles and lift his legs whilst, at the same time, positioning one foot over his sacrum and your toes just touching his lower lumbar area. Apply light pressure only. Give the maximum lift that will stretch the front of his thighs effectively without causing discomfort. Hold this position for about thirty seconds.

HEALING BENEFITS

• *This technique gives the hip joints a rather greater backward rotation than they would normally experience. It aids hip mobility and helps to relieve sciatic pain.*

20   CROSSED AND LATERAL SCISSOR STRETCHES

The methods used for these stretches are identical to those used for the Crossed and Lateral Scissor Stretches with your partner on his side *(see page 108)* with one small exception: your foot is positioned across his lower spine. Repeat on the other side.

HEALING BENEFITS

As for Crossed and Lateral Scissor Stretches in the side position.

21   KNEE TO CALF PRESS

Sit on your partner's sacrum or lumbar region. The exact position is determined by the requirement that your knees should be able to press into his calf muscles. Grasp the front of his ankles and lift them towards you, positioning your knees so that his calf muscles are pulled against them.

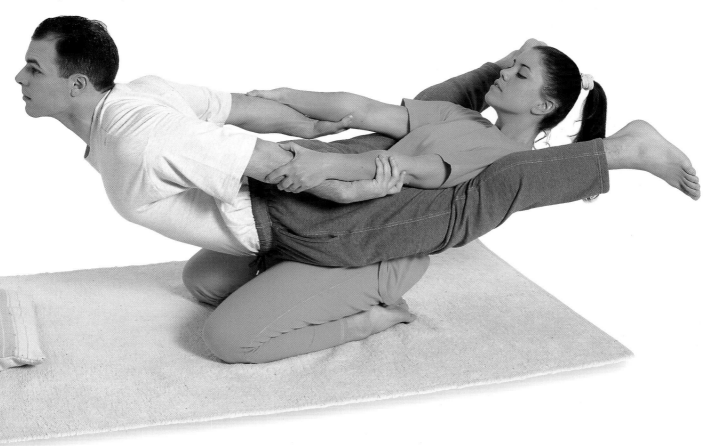

22   INTIMATE COBRA

Kneel and slide between your partner's thighs, lifting them as you go so that they come to lie across the front of your hips. Grasp his arms just above the elbow and have him grasp your your forearms. Lean back with your body weight to lift him into the Cobra position. Hold for at least ten seconds.

HEALING BENEFITS

- *Relaxes spasming calf muscles and improves energy flow in the lower leg.*

MUSCLES STRETCHED & PRESSED

- 19. WHEELBARROW
  Stretched: *Psoas, iliacus, sartorius, rectus femoris*

- 20. CROSSED & LATERAL SCISSOR STRETCHES
  Stretched: *Pectoralis major, sartorius, psoas major, iliacus*
  Pressed: *Erector spinae*

- 21. KNEE TO CALF PRESS
  Stretched: *Quadriceps, psoas*
  Pressed: *Gastrocnemius, soleus*

- 22. INTIMATE COBRA
  Stretched: *Psoas, iliacus, supra- & infraspinatus, serratus anterior, pectoralis major, deltoids, rectus abominis*

Lesson Eight

THE SITTING POSITION

Blockages to the flow of energy between the trunk and the head, such as headaches, are released by the techniques used in this part of the bodywork routine. In addition, tense necks and shoulders are relaxed by the pressing and stretching techniques. Some of the techniques are good for treating 'frozen shoulders' and others manipulate the spine. Refer to Part One Chapter Two (see pages 34–41) for the basic pressing and manipulation techniques. The Sen energy channels shown here represent the upper sections of the Chinese Bladder and Gallbladder meridians respectively. These Sen should be pressed when treating the neck and shoulders in a sitting position.

Sen channels on the neck and shoulders

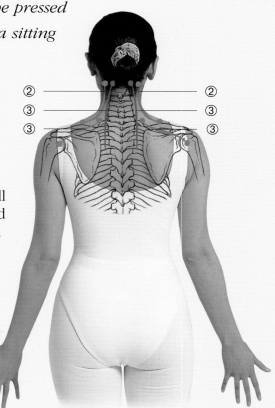

- ② – Starts just below the base of the skull one finger-width to the side of the midline and passes down either side of the spine between the scapulae.
- ③ – Starts on either side of the spine in the large depressions immediately below the base of the skull and continues down the top of the shoulders between cervical vertebra 7 and the back corner of the shoulder joint.
- ③ – Starts on the outer little finger, passes up the back of the armpit to below the outer end of the shoulder, zig zags over the scapula spine and runs up the side of the neck.

ABOVE: *The Sen channels on the neck and shoulder are: ② – Chinese Bladder meridian and ③ – the Chinese Gallbladder meridian.*

1   PRESSING THE SHOULDERS

Touch Method One: Palmar Pressing With your palms placed over the top of your partner's shoulders on either side of her neck, press progressively down her shoulders using the heels of your hands. Pressing should be slow and sustained for up to thirty seconds. Gradually increase the pressure by leaning into the presses.

HEALING BENEFITS

• *Energy flow through the shoulder region is greatly improved which relaxes the neck. Headaches, as well as pre-menstrual tension and pain in the shoulder region, can be eased.*

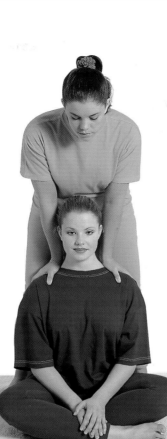

Touch Method Two: Thumb Pressing (inset) Thumb press along the tops of your partner's shoulders along the upper scapula and on the soft tissue on either side of the spine. As you press, feel for any areas of knotted tissue.

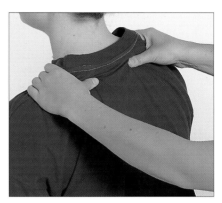

2   ROLLING THE SHOULDERS WITH THE FOREARMS

Place your forearms on top of your partner's shoulders so that they are positioned directly against her neck and, using your body weight, roll your forearms outwards. Move progressively down to the outer margin of the shoulders.

HEALING BENEFITS

• *This technique reinforces all the benefits of the previous exercise.*

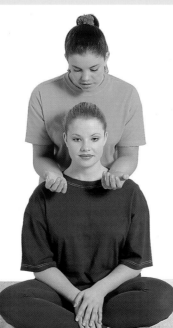

MUSCLES STRETCHED & PRESSED

• 1. PRESSING THE SHOULDERS
Pressed: *Trapezius, levator scapulae, erector spinae, rhomboideus major and minor*

• 2. ROLLING THE SHOULDERS WITH THE FOREARMS
Pressed: *Trapezius, levator scapulae, erector spinae*

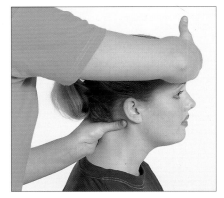

3   THUMB PRESSING THE NECK

Support your partner's forehead lightly with one hand while using the other to thumb and finger press the muscles on either side of her spine. Use a squeezing action. Work from the base of the neck up to the region just below the skull. Swap hands to treat the other side. Repeat at least four times.

HEALING BENEFITS

• *Improves energy flow in the neck channels and is good for treating cervical spondylitis, tense neck muscles, headaches and migraines.*

4   INTERLOCKED HAND/NECK PRESS

Tilt your partner's head forward, interlock the fingers of both hands and thumb press with a pincer-like action up and down her neck on both sides of the spine. Gradually increase the space between the thumbs to progressively embrace those muscles that are further away from the mid-line.

HEALING BENEFITS

• *Sustained deep pressure relaxes tense muscles, easing pain and stiffness; treats headaches.*

5   STRETCHING THE NECK & SHOULDERS

Clasp your hands and place your upper forearm on top of your partner's outer shoulder, then carefully position your other forearm against the side of her head just above the ear. Simultaneously press gently outwards using only very light pressure on the head and more pressure on the shoulder. Repeat on the other side.

HEALING BENEFITS

• *Stretches the sternocleidomastoid muscles to relieve tension in the sides of the neck.*

CAUTION!

Take great care not to overstretch the neck. Do not use this technique on the elderly or those with osteoporosis.

6 BACKWARD ARM LEVER

Take your partner's left arm, flex it at the elbow and raise it in a backwards direction, placing her hand on her left shoulder. Use your right hand to hold it in position while your left hand pulls her elbow backwards. When you feel some resistance to movement, hold that position for a few seconds and then release. Repeat on the other side.

HEALING BENEFITS

• *Opens the joint between the scapula and clavicle. Good for easing frozen shoulder.*

MUSCLES STRETCHED & PRESSED

• 3. THUMB PRESSING THE NECK
Pressed: *Trapezius, splenius capitis*

• 4. INTERLOCKED HAND/ NECK PRESS
Pressed: *Erector spinae, levator scapulae, splenius capitis*

• 5. STRETCHING THE NECK & SHOULDERS
Stretched: *Sternocleidomastoid*

• 6. BACKWARD ARM LEVER
Stretched: *Pectoralis major, triceps, latissimus dorsi, teres major & minor, subscapularis*

7   ELBOW PIVOT LEVER

Raise your partner's left arm and interlock the fingers of your right hand with her left. Place the flat of your elbow very carefully on the trapezius muscle on top of her shoulder. Lean in with your body weight. Use this as a pivot as you lift her elbow backwards with your other hand. Hold for ten seconds. Repeat on other arm.

HEALING BENEFITS

• *Aids shoulder mobility and eases neck pain.*

CAUTION!

• *Do not use this pressure on frail or bony subjects.*

8   TWO-HANDED HACKING ON THE SHOULDERS

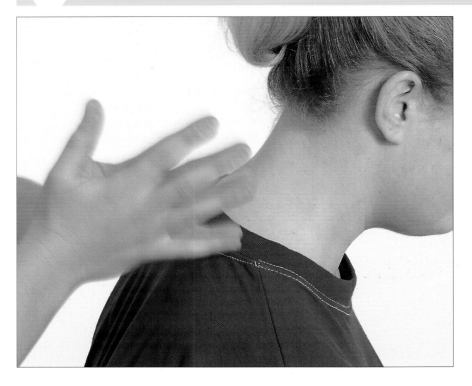

Place both your hands lightly together with your fingers spread apart and touching at their tips. Hack across the muscled areas of your partner's shoulders and between her shoulder blades.

HEALING BENEFITS

• *Hacking has a soothing effect, leaving the shoulders and upper back feeling very relaxed.*

9   THUMBING THE SHOULDERS WITH ARM LOCK

Place your partner's left arm behind her back and hold her hand in position with your right knee. Thumb press up and down the muscled area along the inner border of the shoulder blade. Use your left hand to draw her shoulder back with each thumb press. Repeat on the other arm.

HEALING BENEFITS

• *Eases neck and shoulder stiffness and pain.*

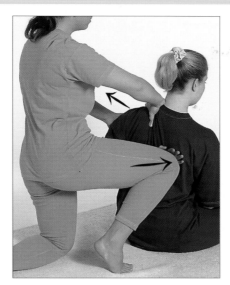

MUSCLES STRETCHED & PRESSED

• **7. ELBOW PIVOT LEVER**
Stretched: *Pectoralis major, latissimus dorsi, subscapularis, teres major & minor, deltoid, triceps, infra- & supraspinatus*
Pressed: *Trapezius*

• **8. TWO-HANDED HACKING ON THE SHOULDERS**
Pressed: *Trapezius*

• **9. THUMBING THE SHOULDERS WITH ARM LOCK**
Stretched: *Pectoralis major*
Pressed: *Infra- & supraspinatus*

• **10. SEATED LATERAL ARM LEVER**
Stretched: *Sternocleidomastoid, trapezius, levator scapulae, teres major & minor, erector spinae, subscapularis, quadratus lumborum, latissimus dorsi*

10   SEATED LATERAL ARM LEVER

Kneel with your left knee resting lightly across your partner's thigh. Place her left palm against the side of her head and grasp her elbow. Let her other arm rest across your thigh and grasp her right shoulder so that it is well supported. Now push her left elbow to create strong lateral flexion of the neck and trunk towards the right side. Hold for a few seconds and then repeat this technique on the other side.

HEALING BENEFITS

• *Improves lateral flexibility of the spine and eases neck pain and tension. Effectively stretches the muscles down the side of the trunk.*

11 SITTING SPINAL TWIST

Using her left arm for support, your partner sits with her left leg across her right. Use your left foot to lightly hold her left foot in place. Simultaneously pull her right arm and push her left knee to generate a good spinal twist. Repeat on the other side.

HEALING BENEFITS

• *Imposes a strong twist on the back, improving spinal mobility and easing lower back pain.*

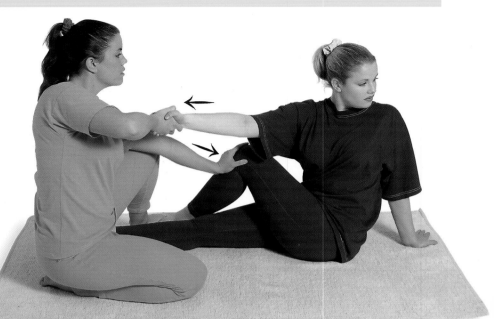

12 PRESSING HEAD TO KNEES

Push your partner's upper body slowly forward until a point of strong resistance is felt. Flexible subjects will be able to touch their knees with their head. Now palm press and pummel on either side of her spine. You can repeat this technique with your partner in the cross-legged position.

HEALING BENEFITS

• *Improves forward flexibility of spine; invigorates internal organs.*

13   BUTTERFLY SHOULDER STRETCH

Ask your partner to clasp her hands behind her neck. Place your forearms against the front of hers and then draw them slightly upwards and backwards to create a strong shoulder stretch. Hold for several seconds as far as is comfortable without causing pain.

HEALING BENEFITS

• *Releases tension in the shoulder muscles and applies a small amount of traction to the upper spine. The clavicular joints (clavicle and sternum, and clavicle and scapula) are stretched and shoulder mobility is improved.*

MUSCLES STRETCHED & PRESSED

- 11. SITTING SPINAL TWIST
  Stretched: *Biceps, latissimus dorsi, trapezius, rhomboideus, piriformis, tensor fasciae latae*

- 12. PRESSING HEAD TO KNEES
  Stretched: *Erector spinae*
  Pressed: *Erector spinae*

- 13. BUTTERFLY SHOULDER STRETCH
  Stretched: *Pectoralis major, Latissimus dorsi, teres major & minor, infra- & supraspinatus, triceps, deltoid, subscapularis*

- 14. BUTTERFLY MANIPULATION
  Stretched: *Erector spinae (neck & back), quadratus lumborum*

14   BUTTERFLY MANIPULATION

Touch Method One With your partner's hands clasped behind her head, tuck your hands under her upper arms and grasp over her hands. Press to guide her into a forward bend in the mid-line. Hold the position for a few seconds. Repeat several times.

Touch Method Two Repeat as above but this time direct your partner's head first towards one knee and then to the other to give a spinal twist.

HEALING BENEFITS

• *Improves spinal mobility and flexibility, and eases lower back and neck pain and tension.*

CAUTION!

Do not force your partner beyond the point where resistance is felt. Some people are very stiff when bending in this direction and a small degree of flexion is adequate.

15   BUTTERFLY SPINAL TWIST MANIPULATION

Retain the same hold on your partner as in the previous technique, but this time place your left knee on her left thigh to hold it in place. Then turn her upper body carefully and slowly to the right to give a powerful spinal twist. Take great care not to overstretch.

CAUTION!

Do not force your partner beyond the point where resistance is felt. Some people are very stiff when twisting sideways and a small degree of flexion is adequate.

HEALING BENEFITS

• *Gives a twist to the spine and eases lower back pain lateral to the main spinal muscles.*

16   FEET TO BACK STRETCH

Sit behind your partner and grasp her wrists. Place your feet on her back on either side of her spine with your toes level with the lower tips of her shoulder blades. Pull on her arms and press with your feet to create a strong backward shoulder stretch. You can take tiny alternating steps down the back to the lumbar region.

HEALING BENEFITS

• *Opens the joints between the clavicle and scapula, and also the clavicle and sternum. Energy flow in the channels on either side of the spine is stimulated to ease stiffness and pain in the lower back.*

17 BUTTERFLY BACKWARD MANIPULATION

Interlock your partner's hands behind her neck, and slide your hands under her armpits, placing your fingers against her forearms. Put your knees against her back just below her shoulder blades and press them into her back against a gentle resistance from your arms. Repeat several times, moving your knees a little further each time.

HEALING BENEFITS

• *Eases upper back pain, improves flexibility; also relieves tension in the shoulders.*

18 CROSSED UPPER ARM BACK MANIPULATION

Cross your partner's arms in front and grasp her right elbow with your left hand and her left one with your right hand. Place your knees mid-back on either side of her spine. Pull her elbows until her arms are tight across her chest. Press your knees against her very firmly. A cracking sound may be heard. Repeat with your knees at different levels.

HEALING BENEFITS

• *Aligns the vertebrae and eases shoulder tension.*

CAUTION!

Not to be done to the elderly or those with a history of osteoporosis.

MUSCLES STRETCHED & PRESSED

• 15. BUTTERFLY SPINAL TWIST MANIPULATION
  Stretched: *Erector spinae (neck & back), quadratus lumborum, latissimus dorsi, pectoralis major*

• 16. FEET TO BACK STRETCH
  Stretched: *Pectoralis major, serratus anterior, rectus abdominis, biceps*
  Pressed: *Erector spinae*

• 17. BUTTERFLY BACKWARD MANIPULATION
  Stretched: *Pectoralis major, latissimus dorsi, teres major, infraspinatus, rectus abdominis*
  Pressed: *Erector spinae,*

• 18. CROSSED UPPER ARM BACK MANIPULATION
  Stretched: *Triceps, trapezius, rhomboideus, some erector spinae*
  Pressed: *Erector spinae*

133

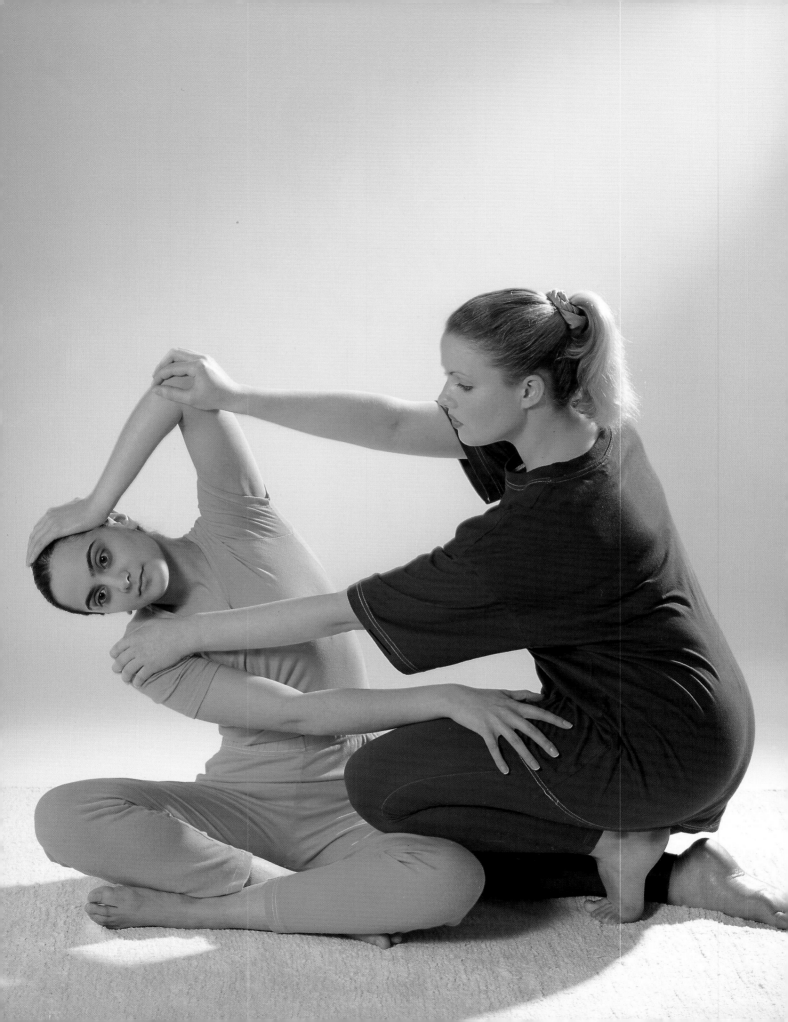

PART THREE

TAILOR-MADE TREATMENTS

Thai bodywork is used essentially as a form of maintenance to prevent pain, rather than as a means of curing it. The spine is very much its focal point because a healthy, flexible spine helps to prevent a wide range of chronic pains throughout life. A high proportion of back-pain sufferers have nothing seriously wrong with the structures within their spine. Their problems are due to muscle imbalance around the spine and weak energy flow through the Sen. When tone in the muscles down one side of the backbone is not exactly balanced in the muscles on the other side, postural defects can arise. These soon affect other parts of the body, such as shoulders and hips, and before long, headaches, sciatica, hand numbness, knee pain and so on, can all develop.

Expert Thai practitioners are able to treat chronic pain of all kinds; to learn their practices it is advisable to attend a training course. However, for those who learn the art of Thai bodywork through these pages, there are some useful guidelines that can help you to handle a partner who suffers from one or other of the most common forms of chronic pain. These conditions are: lower and upper back pain, sciatica, shoulder/neck pain, headaches and hamstring pain.

For each of these conditions, a list of the most effective techniques is given. Accompanying diagrams show specific points where extra, sustained pressing is very effective.

OPPOSITE: *The beautiful shapes that characterize Thai bodywork are apparent in this technique designed to stretch the sides of the trunk and neck. Each move is repeated for both sides of the body.*

CONDITION		POSITION	THAI MANIPULATIONS
Upper Back Pain	This is pain between the shoulder blades. The treatments described here will help to ease this condition.	1. Prone position	Press the whole back, with emphasis on the area above the waist, for five minutes. Now return to the special points indicated for this region of the back and press deeply for five minutes. • All the Cobra techniques *(see pages 118–121 and 123)*
		2. Supine position	• Lifting Head to Straight Knees *(see page 85)*
		3. Side position	• Rotating the Shoulder *(see page 102)* • Rotating the Shoulder with Elbow Lever *(see page 103)* • Stretching Vertical Arm Sideways *(see page 104)* • Pulling the Arm *(see page 104)* • Lifting and Pulling Spinal Twists *(see page 111)* Repeat each of these exercises on the other side of the body.
		4. Seated position	• Backward Arm Lever *(see page 127)* • Elbow Pivot Lever *(see page 128)* • Butterfly Shoulder Stretch *(see page 131)* • Feet to Back Stretch *(see page 132)* • Butterfly Manipulation *(see page 131)* • Crossed Upper Arm Back Manipulation *(see page 133)*
		5. Prone position	Repeat all the presses on the upper back for five minutes.
Lower Back Pain	The following routine will help to ease lower back pain.	1. Prone position	Press the lumbar area either side of the spine for at least five minutes. Pay particular attention to the points marked with a dot.
		2. Supine position	• Rotating the Hips *(see page 78)* • Shaking the Legs *(see page 79)* • Rocking & Rolling the Back *(see page 80)* • The Plough *(see page 80)* • Rocking the Hip *(see page 68)* • Shoulder to Opposite Knee Spinal Twist *(see page 69)* • Stretching the Crossed Leg Horizontally *(see page 69)* • Half Lotus Rock & Roll *(see page 72)* • Vertical Half Lotus Thigh Press *(see page 72)* • Vertical Leg Stretch *(see page 76)* • Bow & Arrow Spinal Twist *(see page 78)* Repeat each technique on the other leg.
		3. Prone position	Whole back pressing for five minutes • Kneeling Cushion Cobra *(see page 118)*

CONDITION		POSITION	THAI MANIPULATIONS
Lower Back Pain continued		3. Prone position continued	• Standing Backward Leg Lift *(see page 113)* • Lateral and Crossed Scissor Stretches *(see page 108)* Repeat pressing of the lower back for five minutes.
		4. Supine position	Repeat the manipulations listed under 2
Sciatica	These techniques will help with the treatment of sciatica, which results from neuritis of the great sciatic nerve which passes down the back of the thigh.	1. Prone position	Press the same areas as those indicated for lower back pain *(see below)* for five minutes.
		2. Side position	Press the entire outer margin of the flexed leg up to the buttock. Press deeply all around the hip joint, then apply extra pressure to the special points for this area *(see below)*. Press for five to ten minutes, then repeat the pressing on the other leg to balance the back. *Both sides:* • All Grape Presses *(see pages 58–59)* • Shoulder to Opposite Knee Spinal Twist *(see page 69)* • Knee to Knee Hip Flex *(see page 106)* • Stretching the Crossed Leg Horizontally *(see page 69)* • Knee Pivot Hip Stretch *(see page 107)*
		3. Supine position	*Both legs:* • Chest to Foot Thigh Pressing *(see page 61)* • Pressing Foot to Thigh *(see page 66)* • 'Tug of War' *(see page 66)* • Vertical Leg Stretch *(see page 74)* • Half Lotus Rock & Roll *(see page 72)* • Vertical Half Lotus Thigh Press *(see page 72)* • Rotating the Hips *(see page 78)* • The Plough *(see page 80)*

Condition	Position		Thai Manipulations
Shoulder/neck pain 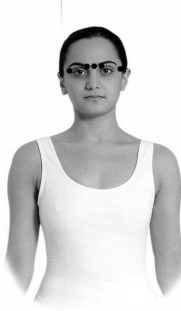	Pain in this area of the body is often due to tension. The treatments described here will help.	1. Seated position	Press and knead the top of the shoulders. Press the special points deeply for five minutes, gradually increasing the pressure. Press and knead up either side of the neck to just beneath the skull. • Backward Arm Lever *(see page 127)* • Elbow Pivot Lever *(see page 128)* • Seated Lateral Arm Lever *(see page 129)* • Feet to Back Stretch *(see page 132)* • Butterfly Shoulder Stretch *(see page 131)* • Butterfly Manipulation *(see page 131)* • Butterfly BackwardManipulation *(see page 133)*
		2. Supine position	• Pressing the Neck *(see page 96)* • Stretching the Neck *(see page 96)* • Pulling the Turned Head *(see page 96)* • Rocking and Rolling the Back *(see page 80)* • The Plough *(see page 80)*
		3. Seated position	Repeat all the neck and shoulder pressing exercises for ten minutes.
Headaches	Headaches are caused by energy blockage at the base of the skull and in the forehead and temples.	1. Seated Position	Press the neck and shoulders in the same way as for the treatment for neck pain for ten minutes *(see above)*.
		2. Supine Position	• Stretching the Neck *(see page 96)* • Pulling the Turned Head *(see page 96)* • Pressing the Face (with emphasis on special points) *(see page 97)*. Choose any of the feet techniques from Lesson One *(see pages 44–51)* to bring the energy down.

CONDITION		POSITION	THAI MANIPULATIONS
Sore hamstrings	Sports injury to the hamstrings is common. The following techniques can be used to treat them.	1. Legs in supine, side and prone positions.	• Palm Pressing *(see page 36)* • Thumb Walking *(see page 35)*
		2. Supine position	• Grape Press *(see pages 58–59)* • Chest to Foot Thigh Pressing *(see page 61)* • 'Praying Mantis' *(see page 62)* • Pressing Foot to Thigh *(see page 66)* • 'Tug of War' *(see page 66)* • Half Lotus Back Rock & Roll *(see page 72)* • Corkscrew *(see page 73)* • Vertical Half Lotus Thigh Press *(see page 72)* • Raised Foot Leg Stretch *(see page 74)* • Vertical Leg Stretch *(see page 74)*
		3. Prone position	• Pressing the Thigh & Pulling the Foot *(see page 112)* • Reverse Half Lotus Leg Flex *(see page 114)* • Intimate Calf & Thigh Press *(see page 117)* • Standing Cobra *(see page 121)*
		4. Side position	• Foot Pressing Thighs & Calves with Chair *(see page 101)*

Regular sessions of Thai bodywork can quickly restore good muscle tone and balance between antagonistic groups of muscles. When this has been achieved, the healthy condition is maintained in a way that only the most dedicated yoga practitioner could hope to equal. The effectiveness of this kind of bodywork is a result of the comprehensive way in which virtually every muscle is treated. None of the muscles – not even the problem ones – can escape attention, provided the full routine for that area is followed.

A Programme for Beginners

For an absolute beginner, the prospect of having to learn the complete sequence of techniques in this book before being able to carry out a complete whole-body massage would be a daunting one. The author has therefore devised this much-simplified progamme that newcomers would be well advised to master before attemptiing one that contains all the most advanced techniques.

• MASSAGING THE FEET
  (see pages 44–51)

• PRESSING THE LEGS
1. Pressing the Inner Feet & Legs (see page 54)
2. Pressing the Left Inner Leg (see page 54)
3. Pressing the Left Outer Leg (see page 55)
4. Pressing the Right Inner Leg (see page 54)
5. Pressing the Right Outer Leg (see page 55)

• RIGHT LEG ONLY
1. Pressing the Leg in the Tree Position (see page 56)
2. Butterfly Pressing the Leg in the Tree Position
   (see page 56)
3. 'Single Grape Press' (see page 58)
4. 'Single Grape Press & Twisted Vine' (see
   page 58)
5. 'Double Grape Press' (see page 59)
6. Pulling the Calf (see page 60)
7. Pressing the Upper Thigh (see page 61)
8. 'Praying Mantis' (see page 62)
9. Rotating the Hip (see page 63)
10. Flexing & Stretching the Leg (see page 65)
11. Pressing the Leaning Leg (see page 67)
12. Rocking the Hip (see page 68)
13. Shoulder to Opposite Knee Spinal Twist
    (see page 69)
14. Half Lotus Press (see page 71)
15. Vertical Half Lotus Thigh Press (see page 72)
16. Raised Foot Leg Stretch (see page 74)
17. Vertical Leg Stretch (see pages 74–75)

• BOTH LEGS & BACK
1. Pressing the Inner Feet & Legs (see pages 54–55)
2. Leg Blood Stop (see page 77)
3. Rotating the Hips (see page 78)
4. Shaking the Legs (see page 79)
5. Swinging the Legs (see page 79)
6. Rocking & Rolling the Back (see page 80)
7. The Plough (see page 80)

• ABDOMEN & CHEST
1. Pressing the Chest, Shoulders & Arms (see page 87)
2. Pressing the Chest (see page 87)
3. Pressing Between the Ribs (see page 88)
4. Thumb Walking the Abdomen (see page 88)
5. Palm Pressing the Abdomen (see page 89)

• SUPINE ARMS, NECK & FACE
1. Pressing the Inner Arm (see page 91)
2. Pressing the Outer Arm (see page 91)
3. Stretching the Arm in the Triangle Position
   (see page 92)
4. Pressing the Tendons of the Upper Hand
   (see page 93)
5. Rotating, Pressing & Pulling the Fingers
   (see page 93)
6. Interlocked Hand Pressing see page 94)
7. Rotating the Wrist (see page 94)
8. Pulling the Arms (see page 95)
9. Pressing the Shoulders (see page 96)
10. Pressing the Neck (see page 96)
11. Stretching the Neck (see page 96)
12. Massaging the Face & Head (see page 97)

• RECEIVER LYING ON RIGHT SIDE
1. Pressing the Back of the Extended Leg
   (see page 99)
2. Pressing the Flexed Leg (see page 99)
3. Pressing Around the Hip Joint (see page 100)
4. Side Single Grape Press (see page 100)
5. Side Single Grape Press & Twisted Vine
   (see page 100)
6. Pressing the Back in Side Position (see page 102)
7. Rotating the Shoulder (see page 102)
8. Pressing the Knee-supported Arm (see page 103)
9. Stretching the Vertical Arm Sideways (see page 104)
10. Pulling the Arm in the Side Position (see page 104)
11. Pressing the Arm Against the Side (see page 104)
12. Stretching the Arm in the Triangle Position
    (see page 105)

Resources

There are, as yet, very few qualified Thai therapists in the West. For a register of qualified Thai practitioners in the UK, or information on Thai massage, Tui Na Chinese massage and acupuncture training courses, write to:

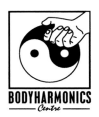

BODYHARMONICS® CENTRE
54 Flecker's Drive
Hatherley
Cheltenham
GL51 5BD   U.K.
tel: 01242 582168

Further reading

Asokananda (Harold Brust). *The Art of Traditional Thai Massage,* Bangkok, Editions Duong Kamol, 1990.

Gascoigne, Richard. The Chinese Way to Health, London, Hodder and Stoughton, 1997.

Gold, Richard. *Thai Massage A Traditional Medical Technique,* Edinburgh, Churchill Livingstone, 1998.

Lundberg, Paul. *The Book of Shiatsu,* London, Gaia Books, 1992.

Mercati, Maria. *Step-by-step Tui Na,* London, Gaia Books, 1997.

Sivananda Yoga Centre. *The Book of Yoga,* London, Ebury Press, 1983.

Thomson, Gerry. *The Shiatsu Manual,* London, Hodder Headline, 1994.

Index

Acknowledgements

AUTHOR'S ACKNOWLEDGEMENTS I am indebted to all my teachers in Thailand and in particular to Chaiyuth Priyasith, Songmuang Khanpon, Pramost Wanna, Wandee Boonsai and Praedik to whom I owe a special thank you. Also, Asokananda (Harold Brust) who kindly gave me the address of Chaiyuth in Chiangmai.

Special thanks go to my husband Trevor for the long hours he devoted to analysing all the main muscles stretched by the Thai techniques, and to my son Graham who studied with me in Thailand. I am also grateful to him and my daughters Gina and Danella for skilfully demonstrating techniques for the photography. Also thanks to my students Alan Orr and Richard Dust, and Shriti Chauhan for additional modelling.

Finally I would like to express my appreciation to Pritty Ramjee and Marissa Feind for their enthusiasm and hard work in designing the book, and to Jane Donovan, the editor.

EDDISON • SADD would like to thank **Trip** / T. Bognar: Bangkok Thailand Wat Pho Temple 6 / J. Arnold: Bangkok Thailand Wat Pho 11, for their kind permission to reproduce their photographs in this book; and Terry Burrows and Phil Hunt for additional editorial work.

EDDISON • SADD EDITIONS

Commissioning Editor	*Liz Wheeler*
Project editor	*Jane Donovan*
Editors	*Terry Burrows, Phil Hunt*
Indexer	*Dorothy Frame*
Art Director	*Elaine Partington*
Senior Art Editor	*Pritty Ramjee*
Senior Designer	*Marissa Feind*
Illustrator	*Joanna Cameron*
Line illustrations	*Julie Carpenter*
Photographer	*Sue Atkinson*
Production	*Karyn Claridge, Charles James*

Thai Massage on Video

This video cassette provides an extensive introduction to Thai traditional massage and demonstrates techniques from the *Thai Massage* manual. It is an invaluable aid in helping you to learn Maria Mercati's unique whole-body routine.

Price £16.99 plus £1.50 UK postage and packing.

Please send cheques, payable to Bodyharmonics Centre, to: BODYHARMONICS® Centre
54 Flecker's Drive
Hatherley
Cheltenham GL51 5BD U.K.
Tel: 01242 582168

• *Overseas orders*: please send an international money order made payable in sterling to Bodyharmonics® Centre, to the value of £22.00. Please note that video cassettes are VHS-format.
• Information on Thai massage, Tui Na Chinese massage and acupuncture training is available on request from the above address.